*An Integrative
Approach*

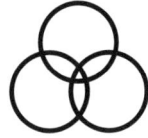

CANCER
An Integrative Approach

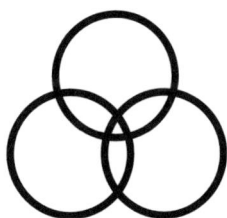

COMBINING CONVENTIONAL
AND ALTERNATIVE THERAPY
FOR TREATING
THE WHOLE PERSON

DR. JOHN A. CATANZARO

WITH ELIZABETH CHAPIN

ISBN 1-929091-01-X
Library of Congress 00-104580

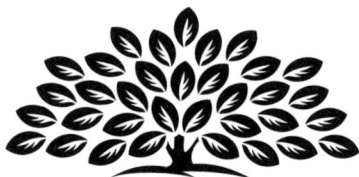

Health&Healing Press™

Health&Wellness Institute, Inc.
5603 - 230th Street S.W.
Mountlake Terrace, WA 98043

www.ehealthandhealing.com

For book orders: 1.800.862.4811

Warning - disclaimer

This material is published for the purpose of information and
education. The information presented herein is in no way intended
as a substitute for proper medical treatment and/or medical
counseling. The author is not liable for the misconception or
misuse of the information provided. This material is not intended
to replace the services of a physician. It is not meant to diagnose
and/or treat illness, disease, or other medical problems and should
not be substituted for professional medical treatment. It is essential
that you remain under the care of a physician.

Printed in Canada

Dedicated to Anna, my companion in life, for her continued love, support, and stability, and to all my children for their love. And to all my friends who have prayed and cared— you know who you are—blessings to you all!

Special thanks to my co-writer, Elizabeth, for her expertise, talent, and valuable guidance. Your labors are much appreciated!

Table of Contents

The Natural Approach Series

The doctor of the future is interested in creating an environment that will enhance the patient's health and well-being. The philosophy of natural medicine provides the motion and the substance sufficient to achieve it.

The Natural Approach Series provides information intended to educate and promote a better understanding of specific health topics. The topics are addressed using the principles of natural medicine, keeping in mind the delicate balance and interaction of body, mind, and spirit. Moreover, it is the author's intent to include a forthcoming work on emotional and spiritual healing. Understanding the principles of natural medicine will facilitate a favorable outcome, regardless of the health condition. Below you will find a description of the guiding principles of natural healing.

The Healing Power of Nature

Every person is made up of three parts: the body, mind, and spirit. These three parts work together and have an amazing ability to heal, if given the chance. The Natural

Approach views the physician as a facilitator to enhance the forces of nature at work within us.

View the Whole Person

Although every person is made up of body, mind, and spirit, there is a complex interaction among these three parts. The goal of the Natural Approach is to promote wholeness with balance among the body, mind, and spirit.

Identify the Underlying Cause

Symptoms are a person's warning mechanism to tell us that something is out of balance or seriously impaired. Treating symptoms only may provide temporary relief from an underlying health condition, but the cause of the symptoms remains. It is essential to search for the underlying cause of a disease, rather than simply suppress the symptoms.

This series mainly addresses physical causes that are common in many people. Many symptoms of ill health may also be caused by emotional or spiritual factors. We recommend you consult with a physician who is committed to discovering root causes in body, mind, and/or spirit.

Take Responsibility for Your Health

The primary role of the physician is to facilitate a person's health and well-being. The Natural Approach Series is intended to instruct, guide, educate, empower, and motivate people to take greater responsibility for their own health. Lifestyle, attitude, nutrition, and diet are all essential elements that a physician may include in a natural treatment design.

Health and Wellness

The ultimate goal of natural medicine is the prevention of disease by optimizing the health and well-being of the individual. Total wellness involves the whole person:

- Physical Health

- Mental and Emotional Health
- Spiritual Health

Total health and wellness are a lifelong quest. We recommend you consult with a physician who will guide you in this quest. Along with the services of your physician, the Health&Wellness Institute is committed to teaching you how to live healthy between office visits.

"

While nothing can substitute for the expertise of your own doctor, no prescription is more valuable than knowledge.

C. Everett Koop, former Surgeon General

"

What Is Integrative Medicine?

A harmonious relationship of the human body, soul, and spirit is where healing begins. Healing is a journey that allows the "whole" person to focus on wellness, rather than disease.

Integrative medicine is sometimes considered synonymous with alternative medicine. However, the term *integrative* specifically refers to the unifying of two approaches to healing.

Both conventional and alternative medicine have much to offer in cancer treatment. Bridging the best forms of both medical disciplines allows for a more comprehensive treatment approach. An integrative approach to treating cancer seeks to enhance the healing energies of the body and minimize negative reactions.

This book will discuss the options for the treatment of cancer in general terms. There are many forms of cancer, and the best approach for the best outcome is in taking an integrative approach. In the treatment of cancer, it is essential not to focus upon the disease process or prognosis, but rather focus on healing and facilitating recovery.

Can I Use Alternative Therapy Without Conventional Treatment?

The best approach is the integrated approach: combining the best that both worlds of alternative therapy and conventional treatment have to offer.

I have many patients who ask this question: Can I use alternative therapy (natural methods) alone to fight my cancer? There are no simple answers to this question. I am not in the capacity to tell my patients that they should *not* use conventional therapies to treat their cancer. Any physician who is put in this position is in for trouble. My role as a physician is to educate and instruct and give my patients the tools that they need to make the best informed health care choice possible. Knowledge is truly power in the sense that it dispels ignorance. Explaining risks and benefits of a given therapy, whether conventional or alternative, is essential.

Are cancers healed using natural methods? The answer to this question is yes and no. There are many cancers that have remitted using alternative methods and many that have not. The same can be said of conventional medicine. In my opinion, the best strategy in cancer treatment is the integrated approach: combining the best that both worlds have to offer. That's an easy statement to make in general terms because the challenge begins when you begin to search out the best therapy for your particular cancer. It takes work and the assistance of trusted experts, family members, and friends. You don't fight this battle alone.

The best results in therapy depends upon many factors:

- Type of cancer
- Therapies being used
- Diet and nutritional health
- Discipline and tolerance
- Emotional and spiritual health
- Inner heart sense of what to do

Type of Cancer

There are many forms of cancer, and they all have different patterns and origins. There are also many books on finding the cure for cancer. Some of these can be very misleading and offer false hope while others are very helpful. Cancer is a complex phenomenon that requires a comprehensive understanding. You must realize that there are no "silver bullets" when it comes to treating cancer and that there are many aspects of cancer we do not understand. In other words, it is not as simple as finding the single cure.

Cancer, in plain language, is a word used to describe disorder and the invasion of boundaries, thereby, adversely affecting the health of the whole person. It is extremely risky in claiming to have the "cure all" for cancer. Any health and healing practitioner who claims such would be able to heal the world and assure immortality, and we know that doesn't exist as much as we hope and pray for the one cure to fit all.

What is the best way to approach this complex disease? The answer is four-part:

1. **Minimize potential harm and maximize healing benefits.** The therapies you choose to implement should enhance the body's ability to heal and reduce the potentially harmful effects. It may be necessary at times to use a therapy that has some strong negative effects initially but is highly effective against the cancer. The key is that the therapy should not be implemented at the expense of the individual. For example, chemotherapy, radiation, and/or surgery should be carefully administered, keeping in mind the health status of the individual receiving it. In my opinion, these conventional forms of treatment should never be administered without supportive therapy that addresses nutrition, immune health, and metabolic health.

2. **Utilize the least invasive means as possible.** Again, the most invasive form of therapy should be used as the last recourse if all else fails. The key is to do your homework and search out your therapy. Don't leave that choice with your doctor. Yes, you must draw from expert advice. But the ultimate decision is yours.

3. **Consider the whole (body, soul, and spirit).** Remember that your well-being depends upon a complex interaction between body, soul, and spirit. This trichotomy is what makes you the unique person you are, and it cannot be separated out. It is not as simple as healing the body alone. The medicine you choose should be medicine that ministers to the body, the soul, and the spirit. Cancer affects the whole person, and the therapy you choose should also.

4. **Rebuild, restore, and revitalize.** These three words are

powerful. They all require input. In your journey of healing, there are therapies that take away life. For example, when chemotherapy and/or radiation is administered, the aim is to kill the cancer cell that threatens the boundary of healthy cells, tissues, and organs. That is the nature of the therapy, and it may be the only thing effective against the cancer. However, this is a therapy that takes away life, and there must be a counter therapy that gives life. Rebuilding what has been taken away is essential when it comes to extending life. Restoration is necessary to renew life energy that is required to fight the cancer. There are various ways of doing this. Nature is an excellent way of restoring life energy. Positive prayer is an excellent way of restoring the life energy of the soul and spirit. If you are too exhausted, have a trusted family member or friend pray with you and for you. Revitalize your existence! You may have to learn to forgive and let go. You may discover that worrying never changes anything and that it doesn't pay to keep this as a pattern in your life. There are certain life issues you must transform and develop into new healthy coping patterns that do not adversely affect your total well-being.

Therapies Being Used

Alternative therapy doesn't always equate to being safe. There are many potentially harmful therapies in the alternative realm. I had a patient who came to see me for a chronic cough that she remembers developing after a specific therapy. This therapy is considered to be an alternative to combating allergies and restoring physical strength. She received a series of peroxide intravenous drips. Afterwards, she developed extreme shortness of breath and a cough. Recently, she had a treadmill test to determine the strength of her heart. She had extreme fatigue because her lungs were not responding the way that they should. I believe that the peroxide therapy had adversely affected her and damaged a portion of her lung.

Whether conventional or alternative, great care must be taken to explore the type of therapy, the results it demonstrates, and the benefits and risks of the therapy. The ultimate aim of any therapy should be to increase the chances of survival with the best quality of life possible.

Dietary and Nutritional Health

Diet and nutrition are the keys to good health. What you ingest is important. What nutrients your body is getting on a daily basis will certainly help beat the odds of cancer. In cancer, you may want to consider a "whole foods approach." This type of diet has fresh vegetables, cold water fish, and colorful pigment foods to restore health. Keep in mind that colorful, healthy foods promote healing. Juicing both veggies and fruits that are fresh and organic is something you should consider. If you really want to fight the cancer, a macrobiotic approach that is very strict and requires much discipline may be beneficial. I have heard of many cancer cases that have remitted using the macrobiotic approach. Whatever you do, diet and nutrition are paramount in your fight against cancer.

Discipline and Tolerance

When experiencing cancer, you will find that you must apply a whole new set of rules to live by. Discipline and tolerance are two essential factors that are required for the best outcome. When you are feeling sick and worn out from the whole process and you're tired of being the experiment for the advancement of medical science, it's hard to think of discipline and tolerance. I encourage you to stick with what you know is working, and don't give up. Continue to thirst for knowledge and implement the positive and let the negative go. If you are tired, maybe you just need to rest from the chemotherapy or radiation. Maybe you need to give yourself a break from all those vitamins, and rest. Whatever the case, try to maintain discipline and tolerance, even with some timeouts. It's best for you and your health.

Emotional and Spiritual Health

The Bible tells us that "a merry heart maketh a cheerful countenance; but by sorrow of the heart the spirit is broken" (Proverbs 15:13, KJV). Transform your thinking into terms of expenditure of life energy. More particularly, think of it in terms of soul energy and spirit energy. How do you want to spend your life energy? Realize that there are all types of "energy robbers" popping their ugly heads up to whittle away your most precious gift, LIFE. How do you preserve this life energy? The Bible answers this well: "Keep thy heart with all diligence; for out of it are the issues of life." What are the issues of life? There are many and they are varied, unique to each individual. But whatever they are and however you face them, learn to let go of those things that steal your life energy away. Transform your soul and spirit, and renew your desire for living. A good bit of advice is to seek God who knows all things and who made a perfect being fashioned in His image. Turn to prayer, and give your anxieties and fears to the One who can do something about them. Let it go, let it go, let it go!

Inner Heart Sense of What To Do

Go with what your heart tells you. Don't ignore it. I had a patient who decided to treat her cancer just using alternative therapy. She used it for months, and her cancer was progressing and taking her life. She came to me in much frustration and very ill. She was afraid to do any other form of treatment because of the horror stories she had heard. She also had friends who succumbed to the ill effects of treatment. I felt in my heart that if this dear lady didn't do something other than what she was doing, she was going to die. She was not ready to give up on life. She wanted life. I told her that she needed to act on her desire to live. I advised that she consider a mild chemotherapy regimen that has worked very well for her type of ancer. This woman is still alive, and it's almost been an entire year that has passed. She is much healthier than she was and recently came into the office very happy about being alive. We are still working together to help fight off the cancer, but this cancer patient has a new hope for living.

In another case, there was a 4-year-old girl with whom I had the opportunity to consult. Her parents wanted to know the best approach for their child's cancer. They had been to conventional practitioners and alternative practitioners alike. They received some strange advice and implemented several alternatives. They wanted to know from me if I felt that alternative therapy alone in their daughter's case would be enough. I felt in my heart that if some other intervention was not implemented, their child wouldn't have long to live. The parents were fearful of what was to come. I didn't offer this counsel because I didn't believe in the medicine that I practiced. I knew in my heart that this child needed specific health treatment. I suggested that the parents consider bone marrow transplantation. As it turned out, there were two years of constant hospital stays and visits. There was the requirement of having a suitable donor, but there was no one in the family who was suitable. They had to use the bone marrow registry that created an alliance for life with a wonderful woman who continues to be in their family. This beautiful child is alive today. Truly, this is a miracle of God that depended on prayerful counsel.

Just remember to get all the required facts, then **Go With What Your Heart Tells You!**

What Is Cancer?

Cancer has become so prevalent in our world that the term is often used as a word picture to describe anything that is uncontrolled, abnormal, and life-threatening in our society.

Cancer is the second leading cause of death in the United States. Cancer risk increases with age, and it is estimated that two-thirds of all cases occur in people over age 65. Some quick facts about cancer:

- Cancer is an invasive, uncontrolled replication of cells in the body.
- Lifestyle and environmental factors are indicated as being the cause of about 60% of existing cases of cancer.
- Cancer risk is high in individuals who have family members with cancer.
- Most cancers require several years to develop.
- If the cancer is detected early and properly treated, most cancer patients have a favorable outcome. But, since cancer can be deadly, prevention should become a way of life.

What Causes Cancer?

Currently, it is thought that cancer is caused by multiple factors. Many physicians agree that cancer has multiple interacting causes. This is contrary to the scientific view of identifying single precipitating factors—such as genes or infectious organisms. Practitioners of integrative medicine know there is no single cause for cancer, nor is there a single cure.

Cancer is caused by a gradual toxic systemic exposure and weakening of body systems (i.e. immune system). However, there are contributing factors which will be reviewed briefly and are listed below:

- Chronic Stress
- Diet and nutritional deficiencies
- Environmental toxins
- Excess exposure to sunlight
- Food additives
- Free radicals
- Genetic predisposition
- Heavy metal toxicity (mercury, arsenic, lead, etc.)
- Hormonal dysfunction
- Immune-suppressive drugs
- Intestinal toxicity and digestive imbalance
- Oncogenes
- Pesticides and herbicides
- Polluted water
- Tobacco and smoking
- Viruses

Chronic Stress

Stress can be defined as a reaction that can potentially upset the function of normal physical and emotional health. There are various causes of stress, such as illness, pain, loss, grief, financial pressures, and so on. Chronic stress directly affects the immune system in a negative way. Stress is part of life and a continual health challenge. The stress load continues to grow with each passing decade. Many Americans today experience stress from the overwhelming job pressures in a fast-paced corporate culture.

Under emotional distress, the brain releases many signals to produce certain hormones that can weaken the immune response. Cancer activity can be accelerated in the presence of these chemicals. Research confirms that emotional stress can increase your susceptibility to illness. Chronic stress that is unrelieved can begin to weaken body systems and suppress vital function.

Diet and Nutritional Deficiencies

The types of foods we eat profoundly influence our health. According to the National Academy of Sciences, 60% of all cancers in women and 40% of all cancers in men may be caused by dietary and nutritional factors.* Some of the negative factors in diet are listed below:

- Excessive intake of meat products
- Excessive intake of processed and smoked foods
- Decreased vegetable and leafy green intake
- Contaminated fish and seafood intake
- Excessive fat intake
- Excessive sugar intake
- Excessive alcohol and caffeine consumption
- Inadequate hydration (not drinking enough water)
- Inadequate essential fatty acid intake (omega 3, 6, and 9's)

Nutritional imbalances may increase cancer risk and facilitate degenerative disease. A wholesome diet with healthy foods is the foundation of good health.

---

*   Committee on Diet, Nutrition and Cancer. Assembly of Life Sciences, National Research Council. *Diet, Nutrition and Cancer.* Washington, DC: National Academy Press, 1982.

Environmental Toxins

There is a continuous challenge to keep environmental pollutants under control. The Environmental Protection Agency (EPA) estimates that as many as 10,000 cancers a year in the United States can be attributed to indoor air pollution. The EPA cannot begin to calculate how many cancer cases are caused by outdoor pollutants. In my opinion, the number of cancer cases caused by external pollutants is seriously high. The key here is to minimize exposure and strengthen the body's ability to defend itself against the negative factors in the environment.

Chronic Sunlight Exposure

Our Earth's protective barrier from UV rays continues to be compromised. The Earth's upper atmosphere has expanded, weakening the Earth's natural shield against it. With this weakening, comes the increase in the number of skin cancer cases that are seen each year.

There are primarily three forms of skin cancer: melanoma, squamous, and basal cell types. Melanoma is the most lethal type of skin cancer. The number of melanoma cases annually is approximately 40,000. The other two forms in comparison are approximately 7,000. Using natural-based protective barrier creams against direct UV rays can minimize the risk of these cancers. Generally speaking, the damaging effects of too much sunlight on fair skin, which can also cause the immune system to be suppressed, can occur years before an actual tumor appears. This cancer risk can be minimized through prevention.

Food Additives

There are many chemicals that are added to foods to preserve shelf life. These chemicals are also used to enhance palatability of processed foods. There are over 3,000 of these chemicals used every year, and many have not been studied for their adverse effects on humans. Some of the most common food additives are: saccharin, cyclamates, aflatoxins, aspartame, and hydroxytoluene. These chemicals are known to cause adverse biological activity, which can increase cancer risk significantly. Eating whole foods that are free of preservatives is the key to minimizing this cancer risk and the answer for healthier living.

Free Radicals

Today, we are exposed to all kinds of external and internal factors that can impair our health. Free radicals are among the most potentially harmful agents in existence. A free radical is an unstable molecule with an unpaired electron that steals an electron from another molecule, producing harmful effects. Antioxidants (Vitamin A, C, E, Selenium, CoQ10, glutathione, proanthocyanadins) are used to protect against these harmful effects. Free radicals are produced by both external factors (environmental pollution) and internal factors (immune defense and metabolism). Antioxidants can profoundly protect against such negative influences.

Genetic Predisposition

All cancer is genetic, in that it is triggered by altered genes. However, just a small portion of cancer is inherited: a mutation carried in reproductive cells, passed on from one generation to the next, and present in cells throughout the body. Most cancers come from random mutations that develop in body cells during one's lifetime—either as a mistake when cells are going through cell division or in response to injuries from environmental agents such as radiation or chemicals.

The involvement of genes in cancer is a complex subject. A term that is now used to describe the family tendency for particular cancers is "family cancer syndrome." The term implies that the cancer is likely to show up in succeeding generations of the same family. Many advances are being made in cancer technology. Many genes are being identified with certain cancer types:

- Breast cancer - BRCA1
- Colon and uterine cancer - BRCA2
- Brain cancer - MSH2, MLH1, PMS1, PMS2

Genetic predisposition doesn't imply that you are going to develop the cancer. It is a term that should inspire you to lead a more health-conscious lifestyle in order to beat the odds of developing cancer.

Heavy Metal Toxicity

Heavy metals, such as mercury, arsenic, nickel, lead, and cadmium, are among the most common known to cause dysfunction in the body. These metals accumulate in healthy body tissue, causing toxic symptoms. Some of these symptoms include fatigue, joint aching, difficulty concentrating, headache, impaired bowel function, and cold hands and feet. There are ways to test for concentrations of these heavy metals. Urinary, blood, and hair analysis are available to determine if concentrations of these are increased in the body. In addition, ELISA/ACT testing is available to give a more accurate result on concentration within cells. Consult your physician on your options. Detoxification and chelation therapy may be indicated to help rid your body of these toxic metals, although identifying the source of exposure is essential.

Hormonal Imbalances

Hormonal imbalance can significantly increase cancer risk. There have been studies that have shown the risk of cancer to be higher in women who are using birth control as compared to nonusers.[†] It is essential to determine the underlying cause of hormonal imbalance and to have the appropriate treatment. Hormonal analyses, using either blood, urine, and/or saliva, are helpful

---

[†]   Weinstein, A.L., et al. "Breast Cancer Risk and Oral Contraceptive Use: Results   from a Large Case-Control Study." *Epidemiology* 2:5 (September 1991) : 353-358.

diagnostic tools. There are other treatment options available. Natural hormone therapy and the use of certain herbs and nutrients demonstrate positive benefits. You may want to discuss this with your doctor.

Immune-Suppressing Drugs

There are a great number of conventional drugs, antibiotics, and vaccines that can have suppressive effects on the immune system. Any suppression of the immune system is unfavorable, except in cases of organ transplantation and tissue rejection. In these cases, it is necessary to modulate the immune system to prevent the loss of function. Vaccinations have suppressive effects on the T lymphocytes, which are an integral part of immune defense and regulation. This could set the stage for the onset chronic disease. Antibiotics hinder immune response and disturb intestinal immune defense by killing off friendly bacteria that protect from potential disease-causing bacteria, viruses, and parasites.

Intestinal Toxicity

Besides the skin, the intestines have the largest surface area contained in the human body. Twenty-five feet of intestine lying out smooth provides approximately 2 ¼ miles of surface area. Many illnesses, including cancer, allergies, and chronic infections, can be attributed to toxic bowel function. If the intestines become clogged and diseased, a toxic environment results. Often, an individual with such a toxic bowel is terribly ill. Diet is an essential part of bowel health. Heavy meat eaters and junk-food junkies are ruining their bowels; and over time, they will pay the consequences. Bowel cleansing and detoxification are strongly recommended. Stool digestive analysis is highly advised to determine the health of the bowel. In addition, replenishing healthy bowel bacteria in order to counteract the potentially harmful bacteria is essential. Speak to your doctor about bowel health and how to optimize it.

Oncogenes

In conventional medicine, the emphasis is to find individual genes capable of causing cancerous cells to proliferate and form tumors. Oncogenes were first identified in the 1970s, and currently there are over 50 different oncogenes responsible for specific cancer types. An oncogene is a gene that causes normal cells to behave in a dysfunctional fashion, thus causing the development of cancer. With the new development that comes from the breaking of the genetic code, some new promising cancer therapies can be designed specifically to attack the cancer and spare healthy tissue. Cancer types will be identified genetically, and therapy will be genetically engineered. The positive benefits may include less side reactions to treatment, better quality of life while undergoing treatment, and hope of cure.

Pesticides and Herbicides

The use of pesticides and herbicides is widespread and alarming. Their usage has increased phenomenally since 1945. Over 400 pesticides are currently licensed for use on our food supply in the U.S. Approximately 1.5 billion pounds of these thousands of varied chemical compounds and formulations are dumped on crops, forests, lawns, and fields annually. The Environmental Protection Agency has identified many pesticides and herbicides that could leave carcinogenic residues on foods. These chemicals build up in body tissue and cause toxic accumulation. This process is called "bioaccumulation." Such accumulation in fatty cells (breast, brain, and sexual organs) can initiate cancerous activity. Detoxification and chelation therapy may be necessary to remove these toxic compounds. In addition, careful selection and cleaning of the foods you eat are necessary precautions to assure healthier body function.

Polluted Water

Our water supply in North America is not as pure as it was 50 years ago. There are many organic chemicals and heavy metals found in higher concentrations with each passing decade. It takes greater efforts to purify the water using reverse osmosis and UV filtration. It is important to remember that approximately 75% of the toxins from water that enter the body accumulate in vital tissues. The liver can become overloaded and impaired by these pollutants, which can, in turn, cause cancerous activity to increase. Another problem is the use of chlorine and fluorine, two toxic compounds used to purify water and assure dental hygiene. Both of these elements are known to initiate cancerous activity. It is recommended that purified, filtered water, without the use of chlorine and fluorine, be used. When shopping for pure water, ask for a chemical and biological analysis. In addition, it is important to know where the water source is coming from. This information is available to you without charge. Your water supply should be free of any toxic elements and/or compounds as well as any harmful organisms, such as Giardia and cryptosporidium, that impair healthy body function.

Tobacco, Smoking, and Alcohol

Tobacco, smoking, and alcohol consumption are among the top cancer causing agents known. It is estimated that 300,000 deaths occur each year in the U.S. as a result of tobacco and alcohol use. There are a variety of cancers that are caused by using tobacco and alcohol:

- Pancreatic cancer
- Liver cancer
- Tongue and lip cancer
- Throat cancer
- Stomach cancer
- Lung cancer
- Leukemia
- Kidney cancer
- Bladder cancer

All cancers caused by cigarette smoking and heavy use of alcohol could be prevented completely. The American Cancer Society estimates that in the year 2000 about 171,000 cancer deaths are expected to be caused by tobacco use, and about 19,000 cancer deaths may be related to excessive alcohol use, frequently in combination with tobacco use.

It would be prudent to abstain from the use of tobacco and alcohol in order to promote a healthier lifestyle. The risks far outweigh the benefits and the medical literature proves it.

Viruses

Viruses are non-living particles that look for a living host to replicate. Approximately 15% of the world's cancer cases have been linked to a viral cause. Hepatitis B and C, human papillomavirus (type 16 and 18), and Epstein-Barr virus are suspect in increasing cancer risk.

Can Cancer Be Prevented or Cured?

Scientific evidence suggests that about one-third of the 552,200 cancer deaths expected to occur in 2000 are expected to be related to nutrition and other lifestyle factors, and could also be prevented. Certain cancers are related to viral infections—for example, hepatitis B virus (HBV), human papillomavirus (HPV), human immunodeficiency virus (HIV), human T-cell leukemia/ lymphoma virus-I (HTLV-I), and others—and could be prevented through behavioral changes. In addition, many of the 1.3 million skin cancers that are expected to be diagnosed in 2000 could have been prevented by protection from the sun's rays.

Regular screening examinations by a health care professional can result in the detection of cancers of the breast, colon, rectum, cervix, prostate, testis, oral cavity, and skin at earlier stages, when treatment is more likely to be successful. Self-examinations for cancers of the breast and skin may also result in detection of tumors at earlier stages. The screening-accessible cancers listed above account for about half of all new cancer cases.

The 5-year relative survival rate for these cancers is about 80%. If all Americans participated in regular cancer screenings, this rate could increase to 95%.

Who Is at Risk of Developing Cancer?

Anyone. Since the occurrence of cancer increases as individuals age, most cases affect adults middle-aged or older. Nearly 80% of all cancers are diagnosed at ages 55 and older. Cancer researchers use the word *risk* in different ways.

Lifetime risk refers to the probability that an individual, over the course of a lifetime, will develop cancer or die from it. In the U.S., men have a 1 in 2 lifetime risk of developing cancer; for women, the risk is 1 in 3.

Relative risk is a measure of the strength of the relationship between risk factors and the particular cancer. It compares the risk of developing cancer in persons with a certain exposure or trait to the risk in persons who do not have this exposure or trait. For example, smokers have a 10-fold relative risk of developing lung cancer compared with nonsmokers. This means that smokers are about 10 times more likely to develop lung cancer (or have a 900% increased risk) than nonsmokers. Most relative risks are not this large. For example, women who have a first-degree (mother, sister, or daughter) family history of breast cancer have about a 2-fold increased risk of developing breast cancer compared with women who do not have a family history. This means that women with a first-degree family history are about 2 times or 100% more likely to develop breast cancer than women who do not have a family history of the disease.

All cancers involve the malfunction of genes that control cell growth and division. About 5% to 10% of cancers are clearly hereditary, in that an inherited faulty gene predisposes the person to a very high risk of particular cancers. The remainder of cancers is not hereditary, but results from damage to genes (mutations) that occurs throughout our lifetime, either due to internal factors, such as hormones or the digestion of nutrients within cells, or to external factors, such as chemicals and sunlight.

How Many People Alive Today Have Had Cancer?

The National Cancer Institute estimates that approximately 8.4 million Americans alive today have a history of cancer. Some of these individuals can be considered cured, while others still have evidence of cancer and may be undergoing treatment.

How Many New Cases Are Expected to Occur This Year?

About 1,220,100 new cancer cases are expected to be diagnosed in 2000. Since 1990, approximately 13 million new cancer cases have been diagnosed. These estimates do not include carcinoma in situ (noninvasive cancer) of any site except urinary bladder, and do not include basal and squamous cell skin cancers. Approximately 1.3 million cases of basal and squamous cell skin cancers are expected to be diagnosed this year.

How Many People Are Expected to Die of Cancer This Year?

This year about 552,200 Americans are expected to die of cancer—more than 1,500 people a day. Cancer is the second leading cause of death in the U.S., exceeded only by heart disease. In the U.S., 1 of every 4 deaths is from cancer.

What Percentage of People Survive Cancer?

Five-year relative survival rates are commonly used to monitor progress in the early detection and treatment of cancer. The *relative survival rate* is the survival rate observed for a group of cancer patients compared to the survival rate for persons in the general population who are similar to the patient group with respect to age, gender, race, and calendar year of observation. Relative survival adjusts for normal life expectancy (factors such as dying of heart disease, accidents, and diseases of old age). *Five-year relative survival rates* include persons who are living five years after diagnosis, whether in remission, disease-free, or under treatment. While these rates provide some indication about the average survival experience of cancer patients in a given population, they are less informative when used to predict individual prognosis and should be interpreted with caution. First, 5-year relative survival rates are based on patients who were diagnosed and treated at least eight years ago and do not reflect recent advances in treatment. Second, information about detection methods, treatment protocols, additional illnesses, and behaviors that influence survival are not taken into account in the estimation of survival rates. The 5-year relative survival rate for all cancers combined is 59%.

Sometimes, patients use statistics to try to figure out their chance of being cured. It is important to remember, however, that statistics are averages based on large numbers of patients. They cannot be used to predict what will happen to a particular patient because no two patients are alike. The doctor who takes care of the patient is in the best position to discuss the chance of recovery (prognosis). Patients should feel free to ask the doctor about their prognosis, but they should keep in mind that not even the doctor knows exactly what will happen.

Doctors often talk about surviving cancer; or they may use the term *remission*, rather than *cure*. Even though many cancer patients are cured, doctors use "remission" because the disease may recur.

How Is Cancer Staged?

Staging is the process of describing the extent of the disease or the spread of cancer from the site of origin. Staging is essential in determining the choice of therapy and assessing prognosis. A cancer's stage is based on information about the primary tumor's size and location in the body, and whether or not it has spread to other areas of the body. A number of different staging systems is currently being used to classify tumors. The TNM staging system assesses tumors in three ways: extent of the primary tumor (T), absence or presence of regional lymph node involvement (N), and absence or presence of distant metastases (M). Once the T, N, and M are determined, a "stage" of I, II, III, or IV is assigned, with stage I being early stage and IV being advanced stage. Summary staging (in situ, local, regional, and distant) has been useful for descriptive and statistical analysis of tumor registry data. If cancer cells are present only in the layer of cells they developed in and they have not spread to other parts of that organ or elsewhere in the body, then the stage is in situ. If cancer cells have spread beyond the original layer of tissue, then the cancer is considered invasive.

What Are the Costs of Cancer?

The National Institutes of Health estimate overall annual costs for cancer at $107 billion: $37 billion for direct medical costs (total of all health expenditures), $11 billion for indirect morbidity costs (cost of lost productivity due to illness), and $59 billion for indirect mortality costs (cost of lost productivity due to premature death). Treatment of breast, lung, and prostate cancers account for over half of the direct medical costs. Insurance status and barriers to health care may affect the cost of treating cancer in this country. According to 1996 data, about 19% of Americans under age 65 have no health insurance, and about 26% of older persons have only Medicare coverage. During 1996, almost 18% of Americans reported not having a usual source of health care. Also, 12% of American families had members who experienced difficulty or delay in obtaining care or did not receive needed health care services.

Cancer Detection and Prevention

Prevention is the most important cancer-fighting tool in existence today.

Cancer prevention should become a way of life, though there are some cancer risks we cannot avoid. Early detection of cancer should be part of overall prevention. There are many cancer detection and prevention tests available. Some of these tests are discussed below:

Cancer Detection Tests

AMAS

AMAS is used for the early detection of breast and prostate cancer. A positive AMAS test indicates that cancer tissue is present in the tissue tested. AMAS is an excellent adjunct to other routine detection testing. AMAS is considered 95% reliable, except in advanced cases of cancer. It is important to remember that testing is always variable and the more accurate it is, the more likely it will detect more precisely. For more information about AMAS testing, contact: ONCOLAB at 1.800.922.8378. This test can be ordered by licensed physicians.

Bone Marrow Aspiration

Bone marrow aspiration or BMA is a diagnostic test that analyzes the bone marrow. This test is done when cancer of the bone marrow and blood is suspected. It is also used to monitor response to Bone Marrow Transplantation. The procedure is invasive and often painful. It can be done under a general anesthetic which cuts down on the pain of the procedure. In fact, I recommend my cancer patients have it done under general anesthetic. The marrow is extracted from the hip and the procedure generally takes about 10 to 30 minutes. Cytogenetic studies can be performed on the marrow sample if requested by the oncologist or hematologist. I recommend that this be done in order to demonstrate the genetic activity of the cancer. However, in some cases, cytogenetic evaluation is not necessary.

Bone Scan

This is specialized imaging for determining cancerous activity in the bone. Bone scan is usually performed using radionuclide techniques. Technetium 99m-labled phosphonates are used to determine abnormalities in bone and joints. The radionuclides are used to minimize the radiation exposure to the patient and are much more specific than X-rays.

BTA (Biological Terrain Assessment)

BTA analyzes an individual's internal environment. This test examines blood, urine, and saliva, and evaluates three criteria: pH (acid-base balance), oxidation/reduction potential, and resistivity. For cancer patients, the test provides more detailed insight into the biochemistry and a more specific treatment plan can be initiated.

CBC and Blood Chemistry

CBC and blood chemistry tests are considered the beginning point in cancer screening. These tests give baseline values and are extremely helpful in finding the cause of certain disease patterns. Again, these tests are used as tools and are not the final word in the diagnosing of cancer. More sophisticated CBC analysis is accomplished by Carbon Based Corporation.

Colonoscopy

Colonoscopy is a procedure that allows the entire colon to be visualized. During this procedure, a biopsy of normal and/or diseased tissue is accomplished. Colonoscopy usually takes about 25 minutes to perform and the patient is given a general anesthetic. It is an outpatient procedure. Colonoscopy is a screening test for cancers of the large bowel. For individuals with increased risk of bowel cancer, it is recommended that this procedure be performed every three years.

CT Scan

Computed Tomography (CT Scan) is valuable in detecting cancer in surrounding tissue and organs. However, some types of cancer may not always show up on this form of imaging. It may be necessary to have more sophisticated imaging, such as Magnetic Resonance Imaging (MRI) and Bone Scan. CT scans are also used to monitor an individual's response to therapeutic treatment.

During the procedure, the patient lies very still on a table. The table passes through the x-ray machine, which is shaped like a doughnut with a large hole. The machine, which is linked to a computer, rotates around the patient, taking pictures of one thin slice of tissue after another. To obtain a clearer picture, the patient may be given a solution of contrast material to drink or get an injection into an arm vein before the CT is done. The length of the procedure depends on the size of the area to be x-rayed. The CT scan is relatively painless. Some mild heat may be experienced if contrast material is used. If you are allergic to certain types of contrast material, notify your physician or technician ahead of time.

Darkfield Microscopy

This type of testing views tiny particles in the blood and blood components. Motion study and cell characteristics are noted in detail with darkfield technology. Darkfield is used to study live blood, magnified about 1,500X, and projects it onto a video screen. A physician skilled in the use of this type of testing can pick up on early signs of illness and design appropriate treatment. Contact Health&Wellness Institute for more information on this type of testing.

ELISA/ACT

ELISA/ACT is a test that was developed in 1984 for the purpose of evaluation of delayed immune response and immune reactivity to certain offending agents. To begin the repair process of the immune system, offending agents need to be identified and avoided. These substances may facilitate further cancer development. This test can help identify and assist the clinician in developing a more effective treatment strategy. Contact Serammune Physicians Lab at 1.800.553.5472 for information on this type of testing.

Genetic Testing

Developments in gene testing are phenomenal. Gene testing examines blood, other body fluids, or tissue for biochemical, chromosomal, or genetic markers for some anomaly that flags a disease or disorder. Gene causation for cancer is an area of continued exploration among cancer researchers. Some inherited forms of cancers are now linked to specific genes.

Heavy Metal Analysis

Continuous heavy metal toxicity leads to both immune and metabolic suppression. A hair analysis test for heavy metal toxicity is a good tool to use since the hair provides a record of these toxic substances. This test is inexpensive, non-invasive, and easy to perform. A 24-hour urine analysis is also useful in detecting heavy metal toxicity, as is a blood analysis.

ELISA /ACT is also used to determine, more accurately, tissue levels of heavy metals because the measurements are accomplished on white blood cells. Chelation therapy (oral and intravenous) is available to detoxify the body tissue. In addition, biological dentistry is also a type of therapy that assists in the removal of mercury and nickel fillings that are known to cause toxicity.

Hemoccult

This test is first line in detecting rectal bleeding that may be associated with colon cancer. This screening test should be given every time you have a major physical exam.

Individualized Optimal Nutrition (ION)

The ION Program is broken down into five profiles that cover specific testing areas. The following briefly describes each of the five profiles:

Amino Acids

Amino acids are the substances of which protein is made. When you eat a protein food, digestive enzymes break it down into amino acids to use for some vital work: brain function, immune system, repair of tissues, energy generation, and blood sugar regulation. Inadequate diets, stress, and poor digestion can deplete amino acids in your body, adversely affecting these functions. It is most often noticed as fatigue. This profile measures amino acid deficiencies in your system.

Vitamins and Minerals

B-vitamins and nutrient minerals are not stored in the body, so we must eat them in our diet. They are essential for converting food into usable energy for many vital functions: nerve transmission, digestion, antibody production, and growth and repair of tissue. For this reason, deficiencies have been associated with heart disease, cancer, and a host of other degenerative processes. In many cases, dietary sources provide inadequate amounts. This profile measures your adequacy of these important nutrients through both organic acids and minerals.

Antioxidants

Normal biological processes and environmental pollutants produce unstable molecules called free radicals that wreak havoc on tissues by setting tiny "fires" of oxidation. This oxidative stress is continual and requires antioxidants, indispensable molecular "fire-extinguishers," to shield against excessive free radical damage. Poor antioxidant protection has been associated with every major disease. This profile measures your free radical activity and levels of antioxidant vitamins.

Regulation of Inflammatory Processes

Fat is necessary for health. Nerve coverings and all cell membranes are made of fatty acids. They produce hormone-like substances that regulate inflammation. They protect against heart disease and cancer, and help our skin, hair, and joints stay young and supple. Most of us have diets rich in "bad" fats: hydrogenated and trans fats common in processed foods. We need more of the "good" fats from fish, flaxseed, and vegetable/nut oils. This profile determines your critical fatty acid balance.

Screening for Organ System Disease Risk

Like gauges in a car, certain chemicals in your body warn of potential problems so that you can make corrections before things get out of hand. This profile uses traditional and newer measures of blood chemicals to detect overt disease or risk of developing health problems. It screens for diabetes, liver disorders, kidney problems, thyroid function, and heart disease risk.

The comprehensive report that is produced for the ION test is a bound booklet containing five sections of information. Section One is a series of graphs showing overall scores in key nutrient-related areas. Section Two is a table of recommended supplementation levels where each nutrient is evaluated from the test results. Vitamins, minerals, fatty acids, amino acids, and other special nutrients are covered. The remaining sections provide increasing levels of detail about your specific test results, including paragraphs discussing each abnormality, pages of laboratory reports, and a glossary of terms so you can look up meanings of the scientific terms.

By applying the ION Program to your life, you can take a positive step in assuring that your body has a daily supply of the high quality nutrients it needs to function best. If you change nothing else in your lifestyle, you have still given yourself an edge toward your personal best level of health and energy. Contact MetaMetrix, Inc. at 1.800.221.4640 for more information.

Mammography, Ultrasound, and Biopsy

A screening mammogram is an x-ray of the breast, used to detect breast changes in women who have no signs of breast cancer. It usually involves two x-rays of each breast. Using a mammogram, it is possible to detect a tumor that cannot be felt. This is a routine form of testing for women over the age of 35 that have a high risk for breast cancer. For prevention of breast cancer, a mammogram is recommended for women over age 40, coupled with a breast self-exam at least one time monthly. Confirmatory ultrasound is a valuable form of imaging that is noninvasive. This should be utilized if mammography is unclear. Biopsy should be performed if the lesion is not clearly distinguished. If there is any suspicion at all, all three diagnostic tools should be utilized along with tumor markers, hormone receptor assay, and confirmatory CT and/or MRI.

MRI

Magnetic Resonance Imaging (MRI) is a sophisticated form of imaging that is even more powerful than the CT scan. In the detection of cancer that affects soft tissue, the MRI is superior to the CT scan. Contrast material can be administered to enhance the visibility of abnormal tissue. For individuals that have a fear of closed places, there are MRI units that are open. MRI is relatively painless. If contrast material is given, there may be some mild heat sensation felt because of the contrast material. If you are allergic to certain types of contrast material, notify your physician or technician ahead of time.

Oxidative Protection Panel

An Oxidative Protection Panel includes a serum lipid peroxide level. Lipid peroxides are the products of the chemical damage done by oxygen free radicals to the lipid components of cell membranes. This oxidative damage, caused by free radical pathology, is thought to be a basic mechanism underlying many diverse pathological conditions— atherosclerosis, cancer, aging, rheumatic diseases, allergic inflammation, cardiac and cerebral ischemia, respiratory distress syndrome, various liver disorders, irradiation and thermal injury, and toxicity induced by certain metals, solvents, pesticides, and drugs. A serum lipid peroxide level, therefore, measures the overall potential for oxygen free radical pathology, the risk for degenerative processes, and the need for compensatory antioxidant supplementation. High serum lipid peroxide levels indicate excessive oxygen free radical lipid peroxidation.

Mechanism Underlying Pathology

This fundamental process underlying pathological conditions demonstrates the widespread application of this concept to many different diseases. Chemically, a substance is oxidized when electrons are removed and reduced when electrons are added. All chemical reactions involve the transfer of electrons. The body generates energy by gradually oxidizing its food in a controlled fashion and storing it in the form of chemical potential energy called ATP. This oxidation process removes electrons sequentially in a kind of bucket brigade, passing the electrons to their final recipient, molecular oxygen, forming water and generating ATP.

Ironically, this energy generation mechanism that is so essential to life can also set the stage for cell damage. The oxidation of foodstuffs is like a controlled fire that liberates energy but can also let sparks fly, giving rise to potential damage. The sparks in this analogy are free electrons escaping the transport system or electrons freed by lack of chain-terminating oxygen (hypoxic conditions). These unpaired electrons readily form free radical molecules that are highly unstable and chemically reactive.

It is these free radical molecules, which rapidly react with other molecules, setting off a chain reaction of radical formation similar to an atomic explosion. The unsaturated lipid molecules of cell membranes are particularly susceptible to this damaging reaction process and readily contribute to the uncontrolled chain reaction. However, other biological molecules are also susceptible to damage, including protein enzymes, DNA, and RNA. Hence, in one process, all levels of cell function may be disrupted. This is why free radical pathology is thought to be such a basic mechanism of tissue injury and end-stage pathology.

It is also clear that environmental agents may initiate free radical problems. The toxicity of lead, cadmium, pesticides, ionizing radiation, cigarette smoke, and alcohol may all be due to their free radical initiating ability.

Role of Antioxidants

To prevent the free radical chain propagation effect, the body uses antioxidants (chemical electron sinks) that quench the biochemical fire. The antioxidants include enzymes such as glutathione peroxidase, superoxide dismutase, and catalase. Vitamins A, C, and E, beta carotene, and coenzyme Q10 are potent antioxidants, which may be their principle role in the body. All these compounds help to control the propagation of free radical pathology in the tissues.

A measure of total serum lipid peroxidation has proven to be a simple, inexpensive, and accurate means of reflecting whole-body free radical activity. This test is presently gaining general acceptance in the research laboratory as a simple, standard means of assessing the body's antioxidant capability or overall oxidative stress. Contact MetaMetrix, Inc. at 1.800.221.4640 for more information.

PAPNET vs. Pap Smear

The traditional Pap smear was introduced about 50 years ago by Dr. George Papanicolaou. This test was designed for the purpose of the detection of cervical cancer. The accuracy of this screening test depends upon the technician's skill in reading the sample. There are many false negatives in traditional Pap smears. PAPNET is better at identifying abnormal cells. The technology improves continuously and offers better scanning and reading of the sample. There are other companies that offer similar technology. Contact: PAPNET at 1.800.PAPNET4 for more information.

Prostate, PSA, and Ultrasound

Prostate cancer is the second leading cause of cancer-related deaths among American men. Prostate-specific antigen (PSA) is a blood antigen that is found to be elevated in cases of prostate cancer, prostate enlargement, and prostate inflammation. If cancer of the prostate is suspected, then the PSA blood testing must be accompanied by prostate ultrasound and biopsy. Adjunct testing, like AMAS, could give a better assessment. Elevated PSA does not always indicate the presence of cancer. The false positive rate for PSA can be as high as 70%. Establishing a baseline is important. A good place to start is as follows:

- PSA level
- Free PSA level
- RT-PCR PSA if indicated
- Prostates acid phosphatase test
- Gleason score
- Other tests and imaging if necessary (CEA, CGA, NSE, testosterone assay, SHBG, MRI, US, etc.)

Some other forms of lab tests and imaging worthy of consideration include:

RT-PCR PSA

This test does not measure the amount of protein in the blood. It identifies prostate cancer cells in the blood, using molecular staging. These PSA-secreting cells are not seen in healthy men. However, they are expected in the blood of men with non-organ confined prostate cancer. This technique is seldom used because of variations of results. With more consistent use, this form of testing is more sensitive and specific because it is measuring on the molecular level. This form of blood testing detects PSA signs in pelvic lymph nodes with more sensitivity than other traditional blood tests. Patients can use this form of testing to establish a baseline and for therapeutic monitoring.

Endorectal MRI

This imaging technique utilizes a long narrow tube that contains radio-frequency coils. This tube is inserted into the rectum while the MRI scan is formed. It gives a clearer picture of the prostate gland and surrounding tissues. It improves the ability to measure the size of the cancer. It detects the cancer more accurately.

MRI

MRI is the method of choice for detecting whether prostate cancer has spread. It is a more specific form of imaging and it can detect soft tissue metastasis very well.

CT Scan

CT scans have not demonstrated favorable results in detecting soft tissue cancers. It is not considered the best choice of imaging for the prostate.

Power Doppler Angiography

This form of imaging is effective in looking at blood vessels and is able to detect blood flow to the prostate. It is able to pick up cancers that are also readily detected by digital rectal exam and

MRI tests. The power doppler is an effective method of detecting early prostate cancer, and it is cost-effective.

For further information on prostate cancer herbal therapy, go to the herbal therapy section entitled PC SPES and read the prostate cancer case study toward the end of the book.

For further information, consult:
The Best Options for Diagnosing and Treating Prostate Cancer by James Lewis Jr., Ph.D. ISBN 1-883257-04-2

The Herbal Remedy for Prostate Cancer by James Lewis Jr., Ph.D. ISBN 1-883257-02-6

Proton Therapy for Prostate Cancer

(Adapted from Loma Linda Website www.llu.edu):

Loma Linda University's Proton Treatment Center is the first proton facility in the world designed for patient treatment and research in a hospital setting. Protons improve physicians' ability to control beam delivery and to treat cancer and some benign disorders more effectively with radiation. More precise beam delivery increases the probability of disease control and reduces radiation received by normal tissues. Unnecessary radiation in normal tissues causes unwanted side effects and limits the use of conventional radiation (x-rays and electron beams). Loma Linda physicians and scientists are specialists in proton radiation therapy, which has been shown to improve control of a variety of cancers and benign disorders. We have proven that protons can be used effectively and economically in a hospital setting where patients can be treated by a team of experts.

At Loma Linda, we use protons for patients who have localized cancers of the brain, eye, head and neck, spinal cord, lung, abdomen, pelvis, prostate, and other sites. We also use protons for noncancerous disorders, such as some forms of macular degeneration of the eye, arteriovenous malformations in the brain, and benign brain tumors. We continually evaluate other conditions and anatomic sites, and are studying ways to combine protons with other forms of treatment.

We investigate, develop, and deliver high-quality proton treatments. We work closely with Loma Linda University Medical Center and Loma Linda University Cancer Institute to support the physical, emotional, and spiritual circumstances of patients and their families. We collaborate with others, such as the National Aeronautics and Space Administration (NASA), to seek better ways to use protons for treatment. In all of our work, we at the Proton Treatment Center support the mission of Loma Linda University and Medical Center: To Make Man Whole.

Tumor Markers

Tumor markers are used to detect and monitor therapy. There are different categories and you should ask your physician for specific details regarding these markers. Some markers are tumor-specific, tumor-associated antigens, hormones, and/or enzymes. When there is any suspicion of cancer, a tumor marker assay can be utilized and is advised. Some common tumor-specific markers are AFP, CEA, CA125, CA15-3, CA19-9, and CA27.29. These tests should be utilized as part of the diagnosis and treatment of cancer. Consult your physician for further information.

Early Detection Test Summary

The following table is a summary of the American Cancer Society recommendations for the early detection of cancer in people without symptoms.

TABLE 1.0 Summary of American Cancer Society Recommendations for the Early Detection of Cancer in Asymptomatic People

Test	Sex	Age	Frequency
Sigmoidoscopy, preferably flexible	M/F	50 and over	Every 3-5 years
Fecal Occult Blood Test	M/F	50 and over	Every year
Digital Rectal Exam	M/F	40 and over	Every year
Prostate Exam*	M	50 and over	Every year
Pap Test	F	All women who are or have been sexually active, or who have reached age 18, should have an annual Pap test and pelvic examination. After a woman has had three or more consecutive and satisfactory normal, annual examinations, the Pap test may be performed less frequently at the discretion of her physician.	
Breast Self-examination	F	20 and over	Every month
Breast Clinical Examination	F	20-40 Over 40	Every 3 years Every year
Mammography**	F	40-49 50 and over	Every 1-2 years Every year

*Annual digital rectal examination and prostate-specific antigen should be performed on men 50 years and older. If either result is abnormal, further evaluation should be considered.
**Screening mammography should begin by age 40.

Biological Therapy and Immunotherapy

The body has a natural ability to protect itself against diseases, including cancer.

B iological therapy (sometimes called immunotherapy, biotherapy, or biological response modifier therapy) is a promising new addition to the family of cancer treatments that includes surgery, chemotherapy, and radiation therapy.*

What is Biological Therapy?

Biological therapies use the body's immune system, either directly or indirectly, to fight cancer or to lessen side effects that may be caused by some cancer treatments.

---

* Adapted from information provided by the National Cancer Institute.

The immune system, a complex network of cells and organs that work together to defend the body against attacks by "foreign" or "non-self" invaders, is one of the body's main defenses against disease.

Researchers have found that the immune system may recognize the difference between healthy cells and cancer cells in the body, and eliminate those that become cancerous. Cancer may develop when the immune system breaks down or is overwhelmed. Biological therapies are designed to repair, stimulate, or enhance the immune system's natural anticancer function.

Immune system cells and proteins, called antibodies, are part of the immune system and work against cancer and other diseases by creating an immune response against foreign invaders (antigens). This immune response is unique because antibodies are specifically programmed to recognize and defend against certain antigens. Antibodies respond to antigens by latching on to, or binding with, antigens, fitting together much the way a key fits a lock.

Immune system cells work against disease, including cancer, in a variety of ways. Immune cells include the following:

- Lymphocytes, the main type of immune cell, are white blood cells found in the blood as well as in many other parts of the body. Lymphocytes include B cells, T cells, and NK cells.

    - B cells (B lymphocytes) mature into plasma cells that secrete antibodies (immunoglobulins), proteins that recognize and attach to antigens.

    - T cells (T lymphocytes) directly attack targeted foreign invaders. T cells direct and regulate the immune response by signaling other immune system defenders. T cells produce proteins called lymphokines, which are one type of cytokine. Cytokines are powerful chemical substances that control a number of cell activities, including the immune response.

- NK cells (natural killer cells) destroy cancer cells by producing powerful chemical substances that bind to and kill any foreign invaders.
- Monocytes are white blood cells that travel into tissues and develop, when needed, into macrophages, or "big eaters," as part of the immune response. Monocytes and macrophages play a key role in phagocytosis, a process by which some cells "eat" other cells and foreign invaders.

Biological therapies, used to treat cancer, target some of these defenses, boosting, directing, or restoring the body's own cancer-fighting mechanisms.

Biological Response Modifiers

Substances used in biological therapies are often called biological response modifiers (BRMs). BRMs alter the interaction between the body's immune defenses and cancer, thus improving the body's ability to fight the disease. BRMs (such as cytokines and antibodies) are substances that occur naturally in the body.

Scientists can now make BRMs in the laboratory that imitate or influence natural immune response agents. BRMs can play many roles in cancer treatment, including directly inhibiting tumor cell growth and acting indirectly to help healthy cells, particularly immune cells, control cancer. BRMs may be used to:

- Enhance a cancer patient's immune system to fight cancer cell growth;
- Eliminate, regulate, or suppress body responses that permit cancer growth;
- Make cancer cells more susceptible to destruction by the immune response;
- Alter cancer cells' growth patterns to promote behavior like that of healthy cells;
- Block or reverse the process that changes a normal cell or a precancerous cell into a cancerous cell;

- Enhance a cancer patient's ability to repair normal cells damaged by other forms of cancer treatment, such as chemotherapy or radiation; and
- Prevent a cancer cell from spreading to other sites in the body.

Researchers are currently investigating a variety of BRMs, and many are being used in cancer treatment. These agents include interferons, interleukins, tumor necrosis factor, colony-stimulating factors, monoclonal antibodies, and cancer vaccines. These BRMs may prove to be most beneficial when used in combination with each other and/or with other treatments such as radiation and chemotherapy.

The Interferons (IFN)

Interferons are types of cytokines that occur naturally in the body. They were the first cytokines produced in the laboratory for use as BRMs. While there are three major families of interferons, including interferon alpha, interferon beta, and interferon gamma, interferon alpha currently is the most widely used in cancer treatment.

Researchers have found that interferons can improve a cancer patient's immune response against cancer cells. In addition, interferons may act directly on cancer cells by inhibiting their growth or promoting their development into cells with more normal behavior. Researchers believe that some interferons also may stimulate B cells and T cells, strengthening the immune system's anticancer function.

The Food and Drug Administration (FDA) has approved the use of a type of interferon alpha for the treatment of certain types of cancer, including hairy cell leukemia, Kaposi's sarcoma (a rare cancer of cells lining blood vessels that often occurs in patients with AIDS), and chronic myelogenous leukemia, making it the first, but not only, BRM approved for cancer therapy. Studies have shown that interferon alpha may also be effective in treating other cancers such as renal cell carcinoma (a type of kidney cancer) and some non-Hodgkin's lymphomas (cancers that develop in the lymph system).

When using interferons, combined with other BRMs or with chemotherapy, researchers are looking for improved treatments for these and other cancers in clinical trials (treatment studies). Investigators are exploring combinations of interferon alpha and chemotherapy to treat a number of cancers, including colorectal cancer, multiple myeloma, and melanoma.

Interleukins (IL)

Like interferons, interleukins are cytokines that occur naturally in the body and can be made in the laboratory. Although many interleukins (including IL-1 through IL-15) have been identified, interleukin-2 (IL-2) has been the most widely studied in cancer treatment.

IL-2 stimulates the growth and activities of many immune cells, such as lymphocytes, that can destroy cancer cells. Lymphocytes stimulated by IL-2, called lymphokine-activated killer (LAK) cells, have proven to be effective in destroying tumors. Lymphocytes can be removed from a cancer patient's blood, stimulated with IL-2 in the laboratory, and returned to the patient as LAK cells, with the goal of improving the patient's anticancer immune response.

Patients with advanced renal cell carcinoma or advanced melanoma have shown the best response to IL-2 therapy. In 1992, the FDA approved IL-2 for treating advanced metastatic renal cell carcinoma (kidney cancer that has spread). Researchers are investigating the benefits of IL-2, used alone or with other treatments, in other cancers such as colorectal cancer, ovarian cancer, and small-cell lung cancer in ongoing clinical trials. Combinations of IL-2 with other treatment methods, such as chemotherapy, surgery, or other BRMs, are also under study. Some scientists believe that IL-2 therapy may help stop certain cancers from growing, which can improve the length and quality of life for some cancer patients. Other interleukins, including IL-3, IL-4, IL-6, and IL-12, are also being studied.

Tumor Necrosis Factor (TNF)

Tumor necrosis factor (TNF) is another type of cytokine under study. Like the interferons and interleukins, TNF stimulates the body's immune cells to fight cancer. TNF also directly affects tumor cells, damaging them and the blood vessels within the cancer. Without an adequate blood supply, a cancer cannot thrive. However, researchers are still uncertain exactly how TNF destroys tumors.

Although TNF has shown promising antitumor activity in laboratory studies, the dose needed for this level of activity is extremely toxic. Researchers have found that TNF therapy is most effective and least toxic when directed at a specific tumor site, rather than administered throughout the body. Clinical trials are under way to investigate the effectiveness of TNF therapy alone and in combination with other BRMs in treating a variety of cancers.

Colony-Stimulating Factors (CSFs)

Unlike TNF, colony-stimulating factors (CSFs) (sometimes called hematopoietic growth factors) usually do not directly affect tumor cells. Researchers have identified several CSFs (such as G-CSF and GM-CSF) that encourage bone marrow cells to divide and develop into various specialized white blood cells, platelets, and red blood cells. Bone marrow is important to the body's immune system because it is the source of all blood cells.

The CSFs' stimulation of the immune system may benefit patients undergoing cancer treatment. Studies have shown that CSFs have the potential to:

- Protect or restore bone marrow function when combined with chemotherapy or radiation, thus permitting the patient to tolerate higher doses of conventional anticancer therapy;

- Aid in separating cancer cells from bone marrow that scientists have removed from the patient's body;
- Stimulate immune system components, enhancing antitumor activity of other therapies; and
- Help treat infections and other problems that may occur in patients who have received chemotherapy or in those whose immune systems are impaired.

Researchers have found CSFs particularly beneficial when used in combination with high-dose chemotherapy. Because anticancer drugs can damage the body's ability to make white blood cells, which are responsible for fighting infection, patients have an increased risk of developing infections during chemotherapy. Doctors must carefully monitor white blood cell levels during chemotherapy. However, using CSFs, which stimulate white blood cell activity, doctors can give higher, perhaps more effective, chemotherapy doses with decreased risk of infection.

Because their immune system has been damaged, people who have had a bone marrow transplant are particularly susceptible to infections after the transplant. Doctors are evaluating the use of CSFs given to bone marrow transplant patients. Researchers have found that CSFs help blood cells in the immune system repair themselves more quickly after transplant, shortening the patient's recovery time and hospital stay.

Monoclonal Antibodies (MOABs)

Researchers are evaluating the effectiveness of certain antibodies made in the laboratory, called monoclonal antibodies (MOABs). MOABs are specific for a particular antigen, and researchers are investigating ways to create MOABs specific to antigens found on cancer cells.

Researchers make MOABs by injecting human cancer cells into mice so that their immune systems will make antibodies against these cancer cells. Researchers remove the mouse cells that are producing these antibodies and fuse them with a laboratory-grown immortal cell to create a "hybrid" cell called a hybridoma.

Hybridomas are like factories that can indefinitely produce large quantities of these pure antibodies or MOABs.

MOABs may be used in cancer treatment in a number of ways:

- MOABs that react with specific types of cancer may enhance a patient's immune response to the cancer.
- MOABs may be linked to anticancer drugs, radioactive substances (radioisotopes), BRMs, or other toxins. When the antibodies latch onto cancer cells, they deliver these poisons directly to the tumor, helping to destroy it.
- Radioisotope-labeled MOABs may also prove useful in diagnosing certain cancers.
- MOABs may help destroy any cancer cells in a patient's bone marrow before an autologous bone marrow transplant in which bone marrow is removed from a patient, stored, and later given back to the patient after high-dose chemotherapy and/or radiation therapy.

MOABs are currently being tested in clinical trials in patients with lymphomas, colorectal cancer, lung cancer, leukemia, and a rare childhood cancer called neuroblastoma.

Because the MOABs originally produced from hybridomas were foreign (mouse) proteins, patients often developed an immune response to them, producing human antimouse antibodies (HAMA). Newer MOABs have been engineered to minimize this problem.

Tumor Vaccines

Tumor vaccines are another form of biological therapy currently under study. Vaccines for various diseases are effective because the immune system can develop acquired immunity to disease after initial exposure to it. This occurs because when T cells and B cells are activated, some of them become memory cells. The next time the same antigen enters the body, the immune system remembers how to destroy it.

Researchers are developing tumor vaccines that may encourage the immune system to recognize cancer cells in this way. Tumor vaccines may help the body reject tumors and also help prevent cancer from recurring. Researchers are also investigating ways that tumor vaccines can be used in combination with BRMs. Tumor vaccines are being studied in treating melanoma, renal cell cancer, colorectal cancer, breast cancer, prostate cancer, and lymphomas.

Side Effects

Like other forms of cancer treatment, biological therapies can cause various side effects, which can vary widely from patient to patient. Because BRMs are often administered by injection, rashes or swelling may develop at the site where the shots are given. Several BRMs, including interferons and interleukins, may cause flu-like symptoms including fever, chills, tiredness, and digestive tract problems. Blood pressure may also be affected. Side effects with IL-2 and TNF can often be severe, and patients need to be closely monitored during treatment. Side effects with antibody therapy vary, and allergic reactions may occur. Cancer vaccines may cause minor side effects, including fever and muscle aches.

Clinical Trials

Details about clinical trials involving these and other biological therapies are available from PDQ, a National Cancer Institute (NCI) database of cancer information. Patients can ask their doctor to use PDQ, or they can call the NCI-supported Cancer Information Service (CIS) to request information about biological therapies and clinical trials.

Immunotherapy

It is important to recognize that immune enhancement therapy heightens immune surveillance. It is essential that the immune system recognizes itself as a friend and not an enemy. This will allow for defense response to the invader rather than healthy cells and systems. There is a communication that occurs between cells and the immune system. This communication is vital and, when enhanced, can improve the environment within the blood and body tissues. The Issels' Vaccine is an example of a powerful form of immunotherapy. There are many immune-modulating therapies that have beneficial effects in cancer treatment. In this book we will discuss the most prominent.

Issels' Vaccine (used by permission)

Josef M. Issels, MD, has become internationally known for his remarkable rate of complete long-term remissions of "incurable cancers" (such as advanced cancers of the breast, uterus, prostate, colon, liver, lung, brain, sarcomas, lymphomas, and leukemias) in patients who had exhausted all standard treatments. After completion of the Issels' Treatment, these patients remained cancer-free for up to 45 years, leading normal, healthy lives. The Issels' Treatment also significantly reduced the incidence of recurrent cancer after surgery, radiation, and chemotherapy, thereby considerably improving cure rates.

The Issels' Treatment was able to reverse chronic degenerative diseases such as arthritis, lupus, Grave's disease, Sjoegren's syndrome, asthma, etc.

In 1951, Dr. Issels founded the first hospital in Europe for comprehensive immunotherapy of cancer. He was the Medical Director and Director of Research. In 1970, the hospital was enlarged from 80 to 120 patient beds. It contained extensive research facilities, including immunological and microbiological laboratories. The hospital's programs included research on tumor vaccines, mycoplasma vaccines, and bacterial vaccines, inducing fever, hyperthermia, etc. Ninety percent of the patients treated at the hospital had exhausted standard cancer treatment.

From 1981 until 1987, Dr. Issels served as an expert member of, and advisor to, the Commission of the German Federal Government in the Fight Against Cancer.

Dr. Issels presented many papers to national and international medical congresses and within programs of continuing education. He also published three monographs.

The Issels' Concept of Cancer Development

The Issels' Treatment is based on the concept that malignant tumors do not develop in a healthy body with intact defense and repair functions. They are present in a specific internal environment that promotes their growth. This environment develops over a period of time due to multiple causes and conditions which persist and remain chronically active even after removal of the tumor (by surgery, radiation, and/or chemotherapy). These remaining causes are responsible for the formation of new tumors which, according to world statistics, occur after local treatment in every second cancer patient.

Therefore, the Issels' Treatment program places equal importance on the removal of the tumor itself and on the causes and conditions leading to the body's tendency to develop malignant tumors.

Pre- and postnatal endogenous and exogenous causal factors can lead to mutagenic, toxic, sensitizing, or neural effects via the transit mesenchyme to secondary damages to organs and organ systems, to functional disturbances of the neural, hormonal, excretory, and defense systems.

These secondary damages, especially the disturbance of the detoxification system, deteriorate the internal environment and can lead to complex metabolic disturbances which are common to all chronic disease and cancer.

Further constant influence of the causal factors and the persistence of secondary damages can produce a functional imbalance and deteriorate the defense and repair mechanisms. Depending on inherited constitution and disposition, this can develop into a chronic degenerative disease and a "tumor-milieu," the ideal medium for cancer cells and micro-organisms found in cancer to grow. The body has acquired the tendency to produce malignant tumors.

With the manifestation of the tumor, the cancer disease enters the recognizable phase. At this time, conventional cancer treatment begins with the weapons directed against the cancer tumor and its symptoms.

According to the concept that cancer starts as a locally confined growth, all measures concentrated on the tumor alone seem causal and exhaustive.

For a detailed chart illustrating this concept, please visit the: Issels website at www.issels.com and read about the treatment program.

Treating the tumor alone is not treating the condition that is producing it: the underlying cancer disease. Consequently, there is a high rate of relapse.

According to the comprehensive concept, however, cancer is considered a systemic disease from the onset and the tumor as its late-stage symptom.

Following this concept, the Issels' Treatment has two lines of approach which are of equal importance and complement each other:

1. A non-specific basic therapy aiming to eliminate the causal factors, repair damages of the early stages, normalize the internal milieu, and restore the immune and repair functions.

2. A specific therapy directed against the tumor itself, such as surgery, radiation, chemo/hormone therapy, hyperthermia, and cancer vaccines.

The **non-specific basic therapy** corresponds with the etiological path leading to the immuno-insufficiency and the cancer disease. It is modified to suit the individual patient's needs. It consists of:

• Elimination of causal factors, such as head foci of infection including dental, alveolar and tonsillar foci, malnutrition, abnormal intestinal flora, fields of neural disturbance, physical and chemical exogenous factors, endogenous and psychological factors.

- Desensitization of the organism which has been sensitized by causal factors by administration of autohemolysates and colloids.

- Treatment of secondary damages, metabolic disturbances, the impaired detoxification and the resulting defense weakness, by general measures, such as hyperpyrexia or fever therapy, oxygen therapy, enzyme therapy, neural therapy, and organ therapy, as well as substitution /supplementation according to individual requirements.

The **basic therapy** is a long-term one without any toxic side effects and aims at the regeneration of the "big resistance," which comprises all the defense zones:

- The extracorporal zone consisting of the physiological obligatory microflora which is responsible for the basic immunity of the organism.

- The epithelial zone consisting of all epithelial surfaces which performs defense, filtration, excretion, and absorption.

- The lympho-reticulo defense zone which performs the important tasks of phagocytosis, antibody production, and detoxification. On this zone, immunotherapy is mainly centered today.

- The reticulo-histiocytary zone, which has been neglected in cancer therapy and research, is the pluripotent mesenchyme embracing almost half of the body weight. It is of great importance to all defensive processes with its various functions:

- the stemcell function;

- the transit function that intervenes between all nerves, organ cells, blood, lymphatic, and intestinal cells;

- the homeostatic function; and

- the defense, detoxification, and storage functions.

These defense zones are successive, are closely interrelated, and are under neuro-hormonal control.

The blockade of only one function of one of these zones, for example, of the excretion or even the blockade of the control system such as the autonomous nervous system, may contribute indirectly to a lowering of the defense potential. During treatment, it was repeatedly observed that by the elimination of head foci, or with a fever therapy, a blockade of the neuro-hormonal functions was broken.

Even in an advanced state of malignant disease, an immune reaction with complete tumor remission can be reached. Holistic comprehensive immunotherapy opens up the following therapeutic possibilities:

- Treatment of cancer of all kinds and stages offering a considerable chance of recovery even for patients in advanced stages who have exhausted all standard treatments.

- Follow-up treatment to prevent recurrence after standard cancer therapy through restoration of the patient's defense and repair functions (the world rate of recurrence is 50%).

- Nontoxic preventive treatment for patients at risk and those with precancerous diseases.

- Preparatory treatment prior to surgery, radiation, and chemotherapy to reduce the risk of complications and, in qualified cases, to render inoperable tumors operable.

- Treatment of chronic degenerative diseases which are untreatable by standard methods.

A system of monitoring regulative functions on a day-by-day basis is an essential tool to determine the effectiveness of the treatment. Therefore, during his 40 years of experience at the sickbed, Dr. Issels developed a system to enable optimum individualized application of the treatment modalities.

Antineoplastons

The most exciting and promising new direction of cancer research is in the body's own natural defense systems against cancer. Dr. Burzynski's work on the development of antineoplastons is both fascinating and miraculous. He has, through the last two decades, made incredible progress in developing this promising therapy. He received FDA approval to enter clinical trials and administer the treatment to selected candidates.

Most cancer experts believe we all develop cancer hundreds, if not millions, of times in our lifetimes. Given the trillions of developing cells, the millions of errors that can occur in the differentiating (maturing) process of each cell, and our constant exposure to carcinogenic substances (smoke, car fumes, radiation, etc.), the laws of probability dictate that mis-developing cells must occur frequently in the life of each individual. It stands to reason that a healthy body has a corrective system to "reprogram" newly-developed cancer cells into normal differentiation pathways before the cancer can take hold.

Cancer cells differ from healthy cells in that they are, in effect, immortal. While healthy cells live a short while and then die, cancer cells continue dividing. The program for cell death is never activated.

Antineoplastons are peptides, small proteins and amino-acid derivatives, found naturally in human blood. Cancer patients tend to have low levels—as low as 2% that of healthy individuals. Antineoplastons work by "reprogramming" cancer cells to die like normal cells. Healthy cells are not affected.

Antineoplastons have a two-pronged mechanism of activity. They suppress the activity of the oncogenes that cause cancer while, at the same time, stimulating the activity of the tumor-suppressor genes that stop cancer.

There are specific peptides that are particularly effective against brain cancer and non-Hodgkin's lymphoma. For further information, contact the Burzynski's Clinic website at www.cancermed.com.

Hormone Replacement Therapy

The best word to describe whether or not hormone therapy is safe and effective in cancer treatment is CAUTION.

There is much controversy over the use of hormone replacement therapy in the treatment of hormone-sensitive cancers (i.e., breast, uterine, and ovarian). Some believe that hormone replacement may be the right choice in opposing the action of the hormone that is causing cancer growth.

In my opinion, it is essential that a thorough examination of hormone activity be accomplished as a part of the clinical workup. In addition, hormone receptor assays give added information as to whether a cancer is expressing a particular hormone. This information is very important because it will help the clinician choose the appropriate therapy.

For example, an estrogen-receptor positive cancer is expressing elevated estrogen activity. This means that the cancerous tissue is positive for estrogen. Giving estrogen in this case would not be a prudent choice. There are cases where a cancer would express positive for both estrogen and progesterone. In this case, neither hormone should be used in therapy. Again, there are cases where the cancer is a nonhormone positive cancer and hormonal therapy may benefit by discouraging further growth. The controversy is: should hormones be used at all in cancer or do they, in fact, demonstrate some benefit? To illustrate this, Web MD had an article on estrogen replacement that can seem quite confusing:

Estrogen Use May Affect Breast Cancer Tumors

by Kurt Ullman, RN
WebMD Medical News

March 31, 2000 (Indianapolis) — Postmenopausal women who develop breast cancer are likely to have a less aggressive kind of tumor if they have previously taken estrogen, a new study suggests. Still, doctors say, the role estrogen medications may play in the development of breast cancer remains controversial.

When women are diagnosed with breast cancer, they are given tests to establish the presence of estrogen receptors (ER) or progesterone receptors (PR) in the tumors. Tumors that are ER- or PR-positive tend to have a better prognosis and respond well to therapies such as tamoxifen.

"We have known for some time that women diagnosed with breast cancer while taking extra hormones seem to have a better prognosis than those who are not," study author Elyse E. Lower, MD, tells WebMD. "In order to evaluate the impact of the biology of the tumor, we decided to look at estrogen and progesterone receptors as a marker.

"Having ER-positive tumors, which we found was associated with extra hormone usage, is a

plus," Lower says. "That may help explain why those diagnosed with breast cancer while taking hormones actually have a better outcome." Lower, whose work was published in Breast Cancer Research and Treatment, is a professor of medicine at the University of Cincinnati College of Medicine.

The researchers performed an analysis of all patients seen by one medical oncologist over a five-year period. Each patient's age, menopausal status, and the ER and PR content of her primary breast cancer were recorded. Patients were recorded as having taken "some" hormones if they had taken either birth control pills or hormone replacement therapy before their cancer diagnosis.

Overall, breast cancers were ER-positive in 72% of the postmenopausal and 57% of the premenopausal women. Most of the patients had taken some form of hormone therapy. Postmenopausal patients who never took estrogen had a lower rate of ER-positive tumors (62%) than those who had (75%). The same relationship was seen for those with PR-positive tumors, which were found in 44% of those who had never used hormones and 58% of those who had.

The difference was not statistically significant for premenopausal women, the researchers say.

"We are not saying that women should be using estrogen because it will make your tumors less aggressive," Lower says. "Before, many women would be worried that because they were taking estrogen their tumors would be worse. Now we know the reason we don't see that is because estrogen probably does make

the tumors biologically less aggressive."

Further research is needed, says an expert who reviewed the study for WebMD.

"Although they have established statistical significance, the clinical significance is not at all clear," Lind M. French, MD, tells WebMD. French is an associate professor in the department of family practice at the College of Human Medicine, Michigan State University, in Lansing.

"It should also be pointed out that the majority of women in this study had ER in the tumors whether or not they had estrogen exposure. We really need a clinical trial before we can begin to make clinical recommendations."

Vital Information:

a. Breast cancer tumors that test positive for estrogen receptors (ER) and progesterone receptors (PR) are less aggressive and more responsive to treatment than those that do not.

b. A new study shows that postmenopausal breast cancer patients who have a history of taking estrogen medications are more likely to have these ER- and PR-positive tumors.

c. One expert says that the clinical significance of these findings remains unclear until further studies are done.

At this time, the best word to describe whether or not hormone therapy is safe and effective in cancer treatment is CAUTION. There is not enough research and conclusive evidence that the efficacy and safety are reliable. However, consider the alternatives. There are natural soy-based hormones that do not exhibit the same metabolic action as the synthetic brands, and there are many herbs that demonstrate phytohormonal properties that may be promising in cancer treatment.

In the realm of appropriate testing for hormonal balance, there are saliva, urine, and blood tests available to give information on fractionated estrogens which include E1 (estrone), E2 (Estradiol), and E3 (estriol, which is known as the protective form of estrogen), progesterone, testosterone, DHEA, and cortisol. It is advantageous to know the levels of these active hormones before initiating hormone replacement therapy. Should you have any further questions regarding hormone testing and therapy, consult your doctor who specializes in natural medicine.

Reduce Breast Cancer Risk

Oral contraceptives have shown to increase breast, uterine, and ovarian cancer risk. The longer oral contraceptives are used, the greater the risk. Other risk factors include family history of breast cancer, smoking, alcohol use, high fat and sugar in diet, inadequate nutrition, stress, and hormonal dysfunction.

How do I reduce the risk factors?

1. Identify the risk factors. Some are mentioned above.

2. Perform proper screening. Self breast exam, mammogram, and ultrasound are effective ways of screening for cancer. These are first line tests that can detect early changes.

3. Improve diet and lifestyle. Eat more fiber and greens, use juicing, eliminate or dramatically reduce the amount of red meat. Definitely be sure it is hormone-free meat. Reduce fat intake. Lose weight if this is a risk factor for you. Practice effective stress reduction and exercise.

4. Consider nutritional and herbal replacement. There are many protective nutrients and herbs that have anti-cancerous properties. Here is a partial list:
   - CoQ10
   - Vitamins E and C
   - Milk Thistle Extract (prevents toxic accumulation of estrogens)

- Saw Palmetto Extract (anti-tumor immune enhancing effects)
- Boron (aids estrogen metabolism)
- Essential Fatty Acids (good fats that aid in strengthening the immune system)
- Calcium D-Glucarate (aids estrogen metabolism)

These are just a few items that demonstrate preventive properties. At the end of the book, there is a case study on breast cancer and a sample treatment plan without listing dosages. This is one among many cases that I have had opportunity to treat in my practice.

IV Therapies

Though cancer is often considered an incurable disease, some treatment plans prove to be powerful and effective.

Intravenous therapy is becoming more popular in cancer treatment. This form of therapy focuses on nutritional replacement, anticancer action, chelation, and detoxification.

The substances usually included in the IV solution are vitamins, minerals, amino acids, chelating compounds, and specialized biochemical medicines that are used to inhibit cancer activity. IV therapy usually takes one to two hours per session and is recommended twice weekly. This therapy is most often used as a complementary therapy, in addition to conventional cancer treatment.

Chelation Therapy

Chelation therapy in cancer is becoming more popular. The rationale behind using chelation therapy is mainly based in detoxification on a cellular level. Dr. Leon Chaitow explains this in his book on chelation therapy:

By now, the concept of free radical damage, resulting in tissue damage and consequent deterioration of circulatory function, should be quite familiar. It is perhaps less apparent that free radical damage is frequently the trigger which leads to malignant changes in previously normal cells. Just as the first benefits to circulation of EDTA chelation therapy were discovered during treatment of heavy metal poisoning, so was the way in which this same treatment could help prevent, and indeed treat, cancer discovered.

Writing in a Swiss medical journal in 1976, Dr. W. Blumen described the strange, but potentially very important, discovery. In the late 1950s, a group of residents of Zurich who lived adjacent to a major traffic route were treated for contamination by lead with EDTA chelation under the auspices of the Zurich Board of Health. These people had all inhaled large amounts of lead-laden fumes and were suffering from a range of symptoms identified as being related to lead poisoning, including stomach ache, fatigue, headache, digestive symptoms, etc. Lead deposits were found to be present in their gum tissues and specific changes were found in their urine, linking their condition with high lead levels.

Some years later, in the early 1970s, people living in the same area were being investigated for the incidence of cancer in an attempt to link the pollution with a higher cancer rate than average. This link was easily established as fully 11 percent of the residents of the road had died of cancer over the period 1959 to 1972, a rate some 900 percent above that expected when compared with people living in the same community but not directly affected by lead pollution. The forms of cancer most commonly related involved the lungs, colon, stomach, breast, and ovary.

But what of the people previously treated with EDTA back in 1959? Only 1 of the 47 people in that group had developed cancer. The cancer rate in people in the contaminated area who had not received EDTA was 600 percent above that of the group who had chelation.

Far and away, the best protection from lead toxicity and its long-term effects is to avoid it altogether. However, this is, of course, not always within the control of the individual and a second best bet is to have the lead removed via chelation as a protective measure against its undoubted toxicity, which can contribute towards the evolution of cancer.

Australian research scientist John Sterling, who has worked at the famous Issels clinic in Germany, mentions in a personal communication that Issels had noted a marked protective effect against cancer after use of EDTA chelation.

Animal studies (using mice) have shown that intravenous EDTA plays a preventive role against cancer, largely, it is thought, through removal of metallic ions, which seem to be essential for tumor growth.

Walker and Gordon believe that the prevention offered to the citizens of Zurich was partly as a result of removal of metal ions and of lead (which can chronically depress immune

*function) and also due to the improvement in
circulation which chelation produced. Tumors
flourish in areas of poor oxygenation and the
increase in the levels of this, which chelation
allows, would, they believe, be sufficient to
retard cancer development.*

*Halstead (1979) points to the significant
increase in metal ions found as tissues age and
the increased likelihood of cancer developing.
There is also a proven link between high levels
of certain metals in topsoil and cancer in the
same regions. Interestingly, he confirms that
most forms of chemotherapy involve drugs
which have chelating effects either directly or
as a result of breakdown of their constituents.
He quotes experimental studies which show
that in some forms of cancer, such as Ehrlich's
ascites tumor, the use of EDTA was significantly
able to strip the tumor cells of their heavy
protective coat, allowing other mechanisms
(such as protein digesting enzymes) to destroy
the tumors.*

*At the very least, EDTA chelation can be seen to
offer a useful line of investigation in cancer
prevention, and possibly treatment, in some
forms of this disease.*

Chelation Therapy. Leon Chaitow, N.D., D.O.

————————————————————99

Chelation therapy is a promising adjunctive treatment in cancer.
The dosage of EDTA administered depends on the height and
weight and kidney clearance of the individual receiving treatment.
Your doctor should calculate the EDTA dose based upon the above
criteria before administering treatment. In addition, the chelation
fluid should include the vitamins that enhance the therapy.
Minerals should be replaced, following the administration of
chelation fluid. Minerals are not included in the chelation fluid

because of the chelating action against the minerals. If it is all given in one lump sum, the individual will not have adequate mineral replacement and can become deficient. Intravenous chelation can take from 1.5 to 3.0 hours to complete, and it is recommended that 20-24 consecutive treatments be administered.

Nutritional Replacement Therapy

Using IV therapy to replace nutritional deficiencies is an efficient method to ensure proper nutrition. This therapy is recommended in addition to conventional treatments. Nutritional replacement therapy offers many benefits to those on chemotherapy who experience a loss of appetite during treatment.

The substances usually included in the IV solution are vitamins, minerals, amino acids, and nutritional and/or herbal substances that enhance immune function. Nutritional IV replacement takes one hour to perform and is generally tolerated well by most patients. For further information on oral supplementation, the next chapter will discuss that and the essential nutrients in preventing and treating cancer.

Nutritional and Diet Therapies

Most integrative treatment protocols begin with consideration of the patient's nutritional balance.

The management of diet includes not only looking at the types of food, but also their nutritional value. This is always a good place to start.

Nutritional Therapy

Nutritional deficiencies can make an individual vulnerable to cancer onset. Today, the food quality is compromised and the concentration of nutrients in food is greatly reduced. When considering an integrative approach to cancer treatment, it is necessary to have nutritional supplementation as part of the overall plan.

Some of the most important nutrients to consider are:

Amino Acids

These are the building blocks of proteins and have specific action in cancer therapy.

Beta carotene

Carotenoids have protective effects against cancer. Vitamin A and beta carotene demonstrate immune-enhancing properties. This nutrient is the precursor to vitamin A. Vegetables (carrots, spinach, and leafy greens) are found to have high concentrations of both alpha and beta carotene. Both forms of carotene are important in nutrition and prevention of disease. Beta carotene has demonstrated useful protective effects in lung and cervical cancer.

Calcium

This mineral can protect against colon cancer. Calcium is essential in the formation of healthy bones and teeth. It is also extremely important in blood clotting and cellular metabolism. The foods that are rich in calcium include dark, leafy-green vegetables, nuts, seeds, and fish.

Chromium

Chromium has been found to be an extremely important trace nutrient in assisting thyroid metabolism and glucose regulation. Immune function improves and a higher resistance to cancer develops when blood sugar levels are regulated properly and balanced metabolic activity is achieved.

Copper

Copper is essential to healthy immune function. Copper is essential for healthy white blood cell and red blood cell activity, and can fight against cancer. However, copper can also accumulate in body tissue in toxic amounts, causing immune suppression and fatigue. Maintaining body balance and addressing the body's needs are the keys to good health.

CoQ10

CoQ10, also known as ubiquinone, is essential to the life of every organism. CoQ10, in amounts of 100 mg daily, has shown to act as a protection against cancer and inhibit further cancer growth. However, CoQ10 is still under investigation as to its direct antitumor effects. It doesn't demonstrate efficacy in all cancers. As a general protective nutrient,

I recommend it. I do not recommend dosing greater than 250 mg daily, unless under the care of a physician. In addition, it is necessary to drink more water while taking this nutrient because of its energizing effect on the body.

Folic Acid

This important nutrient is necessary in proper synthesis of RNA and DNA. It is a protective vitamin against some forms of cancer. Folic acid may become deficient during chemotherapy. Consult your physician on replacement guidelines.

Garlic

Garlic is a food that has been used for its medicinal properties for centuries. Garlic used in cancer treatment can lower the risk of tumor formation in the stomach, colon, lungs, and esophagus. If you don't have an allergy to garlic, then I suggest that you have it in your diet in copious amounts.

Germanium

This is a trace mineral that enhances the availability of oxygen to healthy cells and cancer cells. Cancer cells cannot survive well in an oxygen-rich environment. Germanium slows cancer growth and is recommended in any integrative cancer regimen.

Inositol

Inositol was found to be an important phytochemical that has demonstrated anti-cancer activity. It is classified as one of the B vitamins but really should be classified as a single nutrient. In the body, inositol helps remove excess fat from tissues. It is thought that within this fat accumulates toxins that aggravate cancer.

Iodine

This mineral has shown to be effective in protection against breast cancer. Iodine is necessary in promoting the growth and repair of body tissue.

Magnesium

This is a general protective nutrient in cancer. Your heart and blood vessels need magnesium for healthy function. In addition, magnesium is needed to form healthy genetic material such as RNA and DNA.

Manganese

Manganese promotes healthy oxygen uptake, carbohydrate and fat metabolism, and is important in many enzyme systems. It also has direct action on white blood cells and their binding ability. Manganese is important in regulating a healthy immune system and should be included in the overall treatment plan for cancer.

Molybdenum

This trace mineral is required in small amounts. Deficiency of molybdenum is associated with increased cancer risk.

Omega 3, 6, and 9 Fatty Acids (EFAs)

These are known as the good fats. They are very important in keeping body tissue healthy. According to some studies, these fatty acids may inhibit cancer activity, especially hormone-related cancers. A good, fresh supply of fish, flaxseed, sunflower, and borage oils are recommended for obtaining adequate EFAs. There are also freeze-dried powders available that may be more palatable and can be mixed in juice.

Potassium

Potassium can counteract cancer. By increasing the potassium concentration in the body, enhanced cellular function results, thereby decreasing the formation of cancerous tissue. Dr. Max Gerson found that raising potassium in the diet and increasing its concentrations in the body helped counteract tumor growth.

Probiotics (acidophilus, lactobacillus, etc.)

These are known as the "friendly bacteria" that naturally inhabit the gastrointestinal tract. Probiotics are known to have protective properties against cancer in general. Probiotic activity is the direct opposite of antibiotic action. The antibiotics can wipe out all of the bowel flora. This can leave the bowel vulnerable to more pathogenic strains of bacteria. Probiotics specifically work on the bowel ecology reducing disease-causing bacteria and toxic load, and raising the beneficial bacteria (acidophilus, bifidus, etc.). These beneficial bacteria are needed to provide the delicate balance. Probiotics are known to raise the immune activity in the bowel, thereby, contributing to the overall protection against cancer. Usually as a maintenance dose, I recommend one teaspoonful, 1-2 times daily. In active cancer, when infection is present, I prescribe a therapeutic dose.

Selenium

Selenium is a trace nutrient and is very important in antioxidant defense. Selenium supplementation has demonstrated tumor-inhibiting effects. When taking selenium, prescribed dosing must be followed, otherwise toxicity may result. Doses of 1,000 mcg of selenium have been known to cause loss of hair and adverse neurological symptoms.

Vitamin B6

This vitamin is found in leafy greens, bananas, and other fruit. It is essential for the healthy function of the immune system and overall protection against negative environmental factors such as pollution. It is needed for healthy function of the nervous system and is often consumed in high amounts under stress.

Vitamin B12

Vitamin B12 is used in cases of pernicious anemia, which is an anemia of the blood. Vitamin B12 is necessary for healthy cell development. Chemotherapy and radiation often reduce the levels of B12 in the body tissues and blood. This vitamin should be given along with folic acid, and it is best to give intramuscular injections for better absorption. There are several forms of Vitamin B12. The most commonly used form is known as cyanocobalamin. This form of Vitamin B12 is not metabolically effective. Most patients who have tried this form of B12 say that they really haven't noticed any results.

The preferred form of B12 is hydroxycobalamin, which is long-lasting and metabolically active. Most of my patients notice an immediate energy increase and overall improvement in memory. The next form of B12 is known as methylcobalamin, which is even superior to hydroxycobalamin but also very expensive. I notice excellent results with this form of B12, but use it less frequently because of cost. Vitamin B12 should be included in your cancer treatment plan. The injections should also include folic acid. I recommend at least two injections per week.

Vitamin B Complex

Vitamin B Complex includes thiamin, riboflavin, niacin, and pantothenic acid. All of these B vitamins are important in healthy immune function and glandular support. For healthy formation of body tissue, the B vitamins must be adequately supplied.

Vitamin C

Vitamin C is the most widely studied and has many benefits associated with its use. Linus Pauling's work in the action of vitamin C is a benefit that will be with mankind for ages to come. Vitamin C is an important component in maintaining a healthy immune system and in protecting against many varieties of cancer. The dosing of vitamin C depends upon the individual's tolerance, therapeutic need, and utilization in the body. I recommend to all patients the use of vitamin C in their daily prevention regimen.

Vitamin E

This vitamin is found in dark green vegetables, eggs, herbs, and some oils used in cooking. It is also found in organ meats. Vitamin E is known as a powerful antioxidant. It protects against oxidation caused by free radical activity in the body and strengthens body tissue. There are studies that demonstrate vitamin E's usefulness in protecting against bowel cancer.

Water

Water is an essential nutrient necessary to all living organisms. Water is important in maintaining enzyme systems and detoxifying the body of waste products. A good, fresh purified source of water is a must for every human being. We should be very careful to guard and protect our water, for it is a precious element.

Zinc

Zinc is known as a powerful immune-boosting mineral. Zinc is necessary to have healthy immune function. However, too much zinc can fatigue the immune system. Immune suppression may result if zinc is taken in excess of 60 mg daily. Zinc is an important mineral in protecting against cancer but must be used in proper dosing.

Some other important nutrients to consider are:

Beta-1 3 D-Glucan

This nutrient is considered to be a very potent immune modulator. Some prestigious medical schools, such as Harvard and Tulane Universities, have extensively studied the immune-modulating effects of Beta-1 3 D-Glucan.

This nutrient enhances immunity by stimulating macrophage activity and activating against free radical activity. It is also known to speed up tissue repair and destroy mutated cells that are the cause of many cancers.

This substance is derived from Baker's yeast and is safe to use, unless an individual has an allergy to Baker's yeast.

IP-6

IP-6, also known as Phytopharmica's Cellular Forté, is the one and only patented combination of IP-6 and inositol that greatly increases natural killer-cell activity.

Cellular Forté increases the level of inositol phosphates in the cells. This heightened activity dramatically increases natural killer-cell activity, which strengthens the entire immune system.

When inositol combines with IP-6, they convert into two IP-3 molecules upon reaching the cells. These IP-3 molecules are essential for regulating healthy cell growth.

The IP-6 molecule consists of Inositol and six phosphate groups. When this compound is combined with Inositol (no phosphate groups), IP-6 transfers three of its six phosphates to inositol, creating two IP-3s, once it reaches the body's cells.

In cancer therapy, IP-6 is a potent immune modulator and should be included in the treatment regimen.

Some other important nutrients and immune modulators are:

Colostrum

Colostrum is a nutritional substance that has demonstrated some promising immune- modulating activity. It is the very first substance excreted in mother's milk and essential in laying the foundations of a strong immune system. The product quality varies according to origin of supply and manufacturing standards. In cancer therapy, it may be useful in providing immune enhancement and active immune defense against tumor growth.

MGN3

MGN3 is a powerful immune stimulator that enhances natural killer (NK) cell activity against tumor cells. The research demonstrates some promising results in cancer treatment. For further information on this product, consult www.ehealthandhealing.com.

Diet Therapy

There are many different suggested diets for cancer. Malnutrition is of major concern in cancer patients. Researchers estimate that the cause of death for 40 percent of cancer patients is from malnutrition. Improving dietary habits is an absolute necessity. My suggestion is that you consider reading *What to Eat If You Have Cancer: A Guide to Adding Nutritional Therapy to Your Treatment Plan.* This book is a guide to adding nutritional therapy to traditional cancer treatment programs. It includes an overview of how cancer affects the body, current nutritional information, and meal planning suggestions that facilitate healing.

Another diet you may want more information on is the Gerson Diet. For detailed information concerning this diet, visit **www.gerson.org** on the internet. Below is a segment taken from the *Gerson Healing Newsletter* written by Charlotte Gerson. After reading this excerpt, you will have a feel for the type of diet and therapy that is recommended for cancer treatment.

"━━━━━━━━━━━━━━━━━━━━━━━━━━━━━━━━━

Gerson Patient's Problems

It has frequently occurred to me that, in order to really be sure that the patients understand and follow the Gerson Therapy exactly, I ought to follow them around their house and kitchen for 24 hours. A situation that arose recently amply illustrates the point. I was surprised and shocked by these deviations from the therapy; but, since they were taking place, I felt that it was necessary to share my concerns with our friends and other patients in order to make them aware and prevent errors.

The patient in question was not only very much interested in the Gerson Therapy for his own recovery, he felt so strongly about spreading the word of healing that he organized a Gerson Convention Day. He also invited me to stay at his lovely home overnight so that I could be spoiled with good, organic Gerson food and juices.

The house is located in a wooded area, with beautiful huge trees, at the edge of a small lake.

───────────────────────────

*   Written by Maureen Keane, Daniella Chace (Contributor), John A. Lung. NTC/Contemporary Publishing. ISBN 0-8092-3261-8.

In other words, the air is clean and fresh and the atmosphere relaxing—no problem there. The patient's business is well organized and runs quite well with minimal attention, so he is able to get a lot of rest. There is help in the household, so there are no pressures in the juice and food preparation. But there are at least four major problems in the patient's application of the Therapy:

1. The water is "hard"; it contains minerals. So, like other people in the area, the patient's home is equipped with "water softener" equipment. His very warm, concerned, and cooperative wife is doing everything in her power to help her husband recover. Yet she stated that she brings in "sacks of salt" for the water softener! As our readers know, in the process of removing the unwelcome minerals in the water, the equipment replaces these with sodium. What happens as a result is that the patient washes and bathes in "softened water," loaded with salt. Salt is very easily absorbed through the skin and should never be used by a Gerson patient. Salt is an enzyme inhibitor and the Gerson Therapy is designed to remove excess sodium. Salt is needed for fast growth of tumor tissue. It is also the basis of the "tissue damage syndrome," when normal cells lose their ability to hold potassium while sodium penetrates, causing edema and loss of function. This tissue damage is, according to Dr. Gerson, the beginning of all chronic disease. Naturally, bathing in salt water must be avoided at all cost.

2. We were served a very delicious and attractive lunch, which included a lovely salad loaded with avocados. I immediately asked if the patient, too, was eating them. He was! This

*was another serious mistake, since avocados
contain a fairly large percentage of fat. This is
the reason why they are forbidden, because fats
tend to stimulate new tumor growth! The lady
of the house said that she thought that avocados
were served at the Mexican Gerson Hospital—
which they are not. The problem here is that the
patient or caregiver should not rely on memory.
All these items are clearly set down in* A Cancer
Therapy; *and avocados are the second item on
the "Forbidden" list. We have to ask patients
and caregivers to read and re-read the
"Therapy" Chapter in the book, Chapter
XXXIII, p. 237, and make sure that they
understand all the directions exactly and follow
all instructions.*

*3. Along with the lunch, we had a very nice
vegetable soup. It contained some zucchini,
peas, celery, onions, and a few other
vegetables. The patient asked me how I enjoyed
the "Hippocrates Soup." I had to state that the
soup we had was not Hippocrates soup, as
Dr. Gerson describes it in the book. The
combination of ingredients that are supposed to
be in that soup are clearly described in* A
Cancer Therapy *as well as the* Gerson Therapy
Handbook *(formerly,* Gerson Therapy Primer*),
and they are very specific. Hippocrates (the
father of medicine) understood that this special
combination of ingredients has a beneficial,
detoxifying effect on the kidneys. That is the
reason why Dr. Gerson used it. He felt that this
soup was so important that he wanted patients
to eat the "special soup" twice daily to benefit
the kidneys and help them clear toxins from the
body. Occasionally, one can add extra tomatoes
to give the soup a different flavor; or one can
cut up and roast some onions on a dry cookie
sheet (NO fat, butter, or oil) in the oven. Then*

these can be added to the same basic soup recipe for a tasty treat. However, the basic recipe should remain unchanged.

4. The lady of the house also thoughtfully offered me some enema coffee which I gladly accepted. When I picked it up for use, however, I seriously wondered whether it was the proper strength. I have used enemas for many years and know pretty well what the coffee should look like. This solution seemed too weak to be considered "concentrate" for a dilution of 4 to 1. The lady "thought" that she used the recipe in the Handbook and that it was right. The caregiver must be sure that each enema contains the equivalent of 3 rounded tablespoons of coffee. (See A Cancer Therapy, *p.247.) If a concentrate is prepared, each portion MUST contain the 3 tablespoons of coffee. The coffee enema, too, is so very important that it is imperative that the mixture or solution is correct. Please check and re-check the preparation of the coffee concentrate.*

5. Somewhat less important than the above 4 points: The patient enjoys some bread with his meals—which is quite acceptable. But it is also important to understand that the main requirements for nutrition are the salads, soup, potato, vegetables, and fruit. If all those foods have been consumed, it is all right for the patient to also have a slice of unsalted rye bread. Bread should never be the main part of a meal. Unfortunately, in the last few months, we have had several patients who failed. I also discussed this problem with the most experienced Gerson Therapy doctors: Alicia Melendez and Luz Maria Bravo. Aside from the above, there are other problems we have run across. Let me state here that we (the Gerson doctors as well as myself when I talk to patients) have a serious problem. When we ask the patient about their compliance with the Gerson Therapy directives, even the above patient who made serious errors, will assure us that he is doing everything "perfectly." These patients don't realize what is wrong with their version of the Therapy. When we try to help, heal, and direct the patient on the Gerson Therapy, we rely on the various tools that we have specially created to give the patient and family every possible help and guidance: the food preparation video-tape and the recipe book in the Handbook; the 4-hour workshop tape discussing in detail as much of the treatment as we can; and, most importantly, Dr. Gerson's book. At this point, I need to stress again that the patient must familiarize himself very thoroughly with this material and review it over and over again.

One problem area that keeps coming up is the food preparation. Just boiling the vegetables and putting them on a plate is not good enough. The food preparation tape initiates the cook into various areas to make foods tasty. For example, cooked beets when peeled and sliced can be reheated a little with some freshly made apple sauce and stirred. The vegetable then resembles "Harvard beets." Or, the sliced beets can be dressed with onions, some green pepper strips, and vinegar with flax-seed oil dressing for a beet salad. During the summer months, these salads (also potato salad, string bean or butter bean salad, etc.) are very welcome, refreshing, and stimulating to the appetite. There are many suggested recipes in the back of the Handbook that, I am afraid, are being disregarded. As a result, we often get reports that the patients are weak, losing weight, and doing poorly. Almost always, it turns out that they have "cravings" for pizza, enchiladas, or some other greasy, salty, forbidden food. They are simply hungry because they are not eating well-prepared, healing, nutritious Gerson meals. Gerson meals have another advantage: if the patient (or family member for that matter) eats fresh, organic food, it is truly satisfying. We often get reports that the companions lose their cravings for sweets or heavy desserts. But the key to success is eating tasty food that is prepared with imagination and inspiration from the recipes provided. I must remind patients frequently that when they are on a nutritional therapy, they are on nothing if they don't eat! If patients eat properly, most will gain weight if they are emaciated. Those who are too heavy will lose weight on the same regimen.

Fruits that are in season in the summer, such as cherries, apricots, peaches, nectarines, plums, pears, and grapes are especially valuable— they are high in the best nutrients: vitamins, potassium, and enzymes. Not far behind are apples that are available virtually all year round. Patients (unless they are diabetic or suffer from Candida) should always eat much fruit at night, first thing in the morning, and anytime between meals. One summer food presents a problem: corn. It is perfectly all right to eat fresh corn. The difficulty is that everybody loves corn and during the season is likely to eat it to the exclusion of other vegetables. That is a very bad idea. The vegetables should provide variety and a large selection of special healing chemicals (phytochemicals) and trace minerals. Eating mostly one vegetable is not acceptable and does not fulfill the purpose. Let the guiding spirit of the patient be: "I'll do the best possible to help my sick body heal," rather than "I'll see how little I can do and still get away with it."

From *Gerson Healing Newsletter* Vol. 14, No. 5 (Sep.-Oct., 1999).

━━━━━━━━━━━━━━━━━━━━━━━━━━━━**99**

Another popular diet is the Blood Type Diet.† The basic philosophy of this diet is that your blood type reflects your internal chemistry. The metabolism and absorption of nutrients are different for each of the blood types. The four blood types are A, B, AB, and O. Each of the blood types has its beneficial foods and the foods that must be avoided. This diet is recommended for improving the quality of nutrition and for various health concerns, including cancer.

Other Diet Recommendations

Some individuals seem to do very well following food-combining and acid/alkaline diets.

Food Combining

The basic approach of this diet is to keep your proteins and starches away from each other. For example: having a protein like fish with vegetables instead of fish and potato or rice. It is okay to have pasta (starch) and vegetables. In this diet, melons and fruits should be eaten separately. Nuts and seeds are usually snack meals. The philosophy of this diet is to lessen the load on the digestive tract for better digestion and absorption of the food. I have noticed benefits from this dietary approach.

Acid/Alkaline

In this dietary approach, it is thought that the more alkaline the food, the healthier you will be. Advocates of this diet say that alkalinity equals longevity. There are foods that can

---

† *Eat Right for Your Type.* Dr. Peter D'Adamo. G.P. Putnam's Sons. ISBN 0-399-14255-X.

make your body more acidic or alkaline. The majority of the foods that are alkaline are vegetables and some fruits. Meats, dairy, and some grains tend to produce more acid. The more acidic people are, the more likely they will develop cancer or a degenerative disease.

Juicing

Juicing should be an essential part of cancer therapy. Juicing the yellow, green, orange, and purple pigment fruits and vegetables is very nutritious and immune-enhancing. However, juicing depends upon the tolerance of the individual. If you are really tired and fatigued, you may not have the energy to juice and a friend or relative may have to help you during such an important time in your life. Another important aspect of juicing is that the fruits and vegetables that are selected must be the highest grade in season as well as organic. All of the produce must be washed in an organic food wash before juiced.

An example of vegetables and fruits to be juiced include: apple, pear, blueberry, blackberry, apricot, kale, lemon, spinach, onion, garlic, mustard greens, carrot, asparagus, wheat grass, tomatoes etc. You may want to experiment a bit and combine the compatible flavors. Remember that color and hearty flavor are the key ingredients that make up a healing juice.

I have observed many cancer patients gain energy and some even had their cancers go into remission by maintaining a strict vegetarian diet and juicing. Another option is to add a protein powder to your juice to boost up the protein value.

Immunocal®

Immunocal is a whey-based protein powder isolate that has powerful immune-modulating properties. It is used extensively in cancer to maintain nutritional health and to enhance immune health while a patient is receiving cancer treatment. Immunocal maintains a healthier immune system by sustaining levels of glutathione in the lymphocytes. Glutathione helps to support the proper functioning of your immune system:

- Your body's natural immune activity involving unimpeded multiplication of lymphocytes and antibody production requires maintenance of normal levels of glutathione inside the lymphocytes.
- Glutathione plays a central, protective role against the damaging effects of pollutants and free radicals.
- Without glutathione, other important antioxidants, such as vitamins C and E, cannot adequately do their job.
- The second major function of glutathione consists of the body's natural detoxification of foreign chemical compounds.

There are many patients who have benefited from the use of Immunocal, and I recommend it. However, if there is an allergy or sensitivity to whey, then I would find another alternative.

For further information on Immunocal, you may search their website at http://www.immunocal.com

UltraBalance Medical Food Powders

Another quality product available in cancer treatment is the UltraBalance Medical Food Powders. I have utilized this product and incorporated it into the diet and treatment plan for my patients. UltraBalance Medical Foods are designed to nutritionally support patients with food sensitivities, during detoxification and gastrointestinal support programs, for general nutrition, and during weight loss or weight maintenance. In cancer treatment, it is essential to maintain adequate nutritional intake. I highly recommend this as part of the cancer treatment program.

For further information, contact www.ultrabalance.com

Nutritional Glandular Support

A cancer treatment program that doesn't include support for the glands is not complete. Remember, cancer affects every organ, gland, and system. The glandular system includes the pituitary gland, thyroid gland, adrenal glands, and reproductive glands. All of these glands work together to keep hormone balance. Some cancers may directly involve these glands, making nutritional support imperative. Some nutritional supports to consider:

- Adrenal support formula (should include adrenal gland, pantothenic acid, panax ginseng, licorice root, zinc, and other supportive B vitamins). Some good formula recommendations are Cortrex (Thorne Research) and Adrenoplex (Priority One). Before beginning any of these formulas, consult your doctor.

- Thyroid support formula (should include thyroid gland, L-tyrosine, and thyroid balancing herbs). Some good formula recommendations are Spectra 303-T (NF Formulations) and Hydrotropic PMG (Standard Process Labs). Before beginning any of these formulas, consult your doctor.

- Free-form amino acids
- CoQ10
- Panax ginseng
- Vitamin B12
- Folic acid
- DHEA

Herbal Therapy

Cancer studies indicate that cancer develops when the body's immune system is weakened; therefore, a strengthened immune system is crucial in the fight against cancer.

M any herbal therapies focus on restoring health to the body's immune system so the body can work to fight against cancer. Various herbs are being carefully studied to determine their beneficial use, not only in fighting cancer, but in curing the disease.

Herbs Used in Cancer Therapy

The pharmaceutical drugs found in nature contain significant healing powers. The following list of natural herbs provides a description of the herb, active ingredients, common uses, dosing, adverse reactions, and contraindications.

WARNING*: Natural does not always mean safe. Recommended therapies are only advised under the supervision of your health care provider.*

Aloe Vera

This plant's origin is from Africa. The parts of the plant used are its leaves and roots. The plant produces a gel substance that contains many active compounds. Aloe had been used historically for the treatment of constipation. The root of the plant was used for intestinal colic. Aloe has also been used in India to treat intestinal infections.

Active Ingredients

The compounds aloe contains include acemannan, anthrone-10-C-glykosyls, including aloin A, aloin B, 7-hydroxyaloins and 1, 8-dihydroxyanthraquinones, including aloe-emodin. Aloe also contains flavonoids and resins.

Uses

In cancer therapy, aloe gel can be beneficial in stimulating immunity. In animal studies, a water-soluble compound was found in aloe vera known as acemannan. This compound is a potent immune stimulant and antitumor agent.

Dosing

Criteria for therapeutic dosing has not been established for humans. For constipation, a single dose of 50-200 mg should be taken each day for a maximum of ten days. Topical application of a stabilized gel may be used for minor burns. For more serious burns, a health professional must be contacted before application is made. Internal use of the gel is at 30 ml three times daily.

Adverse Reactions

There have been some reports of allergic reactions to aloe but it is rare. If used as a laxative, aloe must not be used for more than 10 consecutive days. Chronic use of aloe can lead to potassium deficiency, especially when used with licorice, thiazide diuretics, and steroids. The actions of cardiac and antiarhythmic drugs can be affected by the use of aloe.

Contraindications

Aloe should not be used in cases of intestinal obstruction and acutely inflamed intestinal diseases (ulcerative colitis, Crohn's disease), appendicitis, and abdominal pain of unknown origin. Aloe should not be used in pregnancy and in children under 12 years of age.

Amygdalin

Amygdalin is also known as Laetrile or vitamin B17. This substance is concentrated in kernals of apricots. Amygdalin has been used in China for centuries. It has demonstrated strong cancer-fighting potential in general. Amygdalin is given both orally and intravenously. There is much controversy over its use and benefits in cancer treatment.

Arabinogalactans (Larix)

Larix is known as an immune enhancer that is a sweet-tasting powder derived from the Western Larch tree (*Larix occidentalis*). Dr. Peter D'Adamo identified and developed Larix from a paper by-product. The immune related effects of Larix powder include:

- Stimulation of NK cells activity.
- Stimulation of macrophage activity.
- Enhanced tumor cell-killing due to increased immune stimulation.

Larix is available from Eclectic Institute at 1.800.332.4372.

Astragalus (Astragalus membranaceus)

This plant's origin is from China. The main part of the plant used is its root, which is aged four to seven years before use. In cancer therapy, this botanical is very useful for enhancing immune response and in chemotherapy support.

Active Ingredients

Astragalus contains flavonoids, polysaccharides, triterpene glycosides (e.g., astraglycosides I-VII), amino acids, and trace minerals. Astragalus has action on the white blood cells and is used in cancer treatment to restore counts toward the reference range.

Uses

Traditional Chinese medicine uses this herb for night sweats, fatigue, loss of appetite, weakness, and diarrhea. Empirical medicine has used this herb for the common cold, sore throat, and general immune modulating.

Dosage

The recommended dosing for Astragalus is 500 mg, two to three capsules, three times daily or 3-5 ml three times daily. There are no negative side effects known when used as recommended.

Cat's Claw
(Uncaria guianensis; Uncaria tomentosa)

Cat's claw, or uña de gato as it is also called, has piqued many people's interest lately: first, because it comes from remote and exotic rain forests, and second, because it is believed to act on the immune system.

Both of the species referred to as cat's claw are climbing woody vines (lianas) in the Amazon Rain Forest. The name refers to the small sharp spines on the stem, near the leaf, curved back like a cat's claw.

U. guianensis has been used by native people in South America to treat intestinal problems and to heal wounds. The bark is used by different tribes for different purposes: some find it an effective contraceptive, and others use it to treat gonorrhea. This plant is widely used to relieve the pain of rheumatism and to reduce inflammation as well as for dysentery and ulcers. This species of cat's claw is preferred in the European market.

U. tomentosa, from the Peruvian headwaters of the Amazon, is often used for arthritis, ulcers, and other intestinal problems. In addition, it is prized as a general tonic for its "life-giving" properties and is used for certain skin diseases. The North American marketplace provides the major commercial outlet for this species. The bark is the part of the plant generally used for medicinal purposes.

Active Ingredients

Research on the constituents of uña de gato was begun only a few decades ago. Both species appear to contain alkaloids. *U. tomentosa* also contains quinovic acid glycosides and some novel triterpenes.

Uses

Traditional use by Amazonian tribes includes the treatment of a number of digestive disorders. Uña de gato is sometimes promoted in the United States to treat problems such as hemorrhoids, gastritis, colitis, ulcers, diverticulitis, and leaky bowel. These applications appear to be based more on reports of folk medicine from the Amazon than on clinical or animal studies.

In the test tube, most of the alkaloids of *U. tomentosa* can be shown to activate immune-system cells. Several quinovic acid glycosides are active against various viruses in the laboratory. Many of these compounds also counteract inflammation caused experimentally in rat-paw tests.

One important alkaloid lowers blood pressure, relaxes and dilates peripheral blood vessels, slows heart rate, and lowers cholesterol. Another acts as a diuretic. The immune-stimulating effects of *U. tomentosa* have attracted attention for the possibility that the herb might be useful against cancer.

Dosage

One gram of root bark to 1 cup of boiling water, steeped for 10 minutes. After cooling and straining, 1 cup is drunk 2-3 times per day. In tincture form, 1-2 ml, 2 times per day. In standardized extract, between 20-60 mg per day.

Contraindications

Pregnant women should not take cat's claw because its safety and mode of action have been inadequately studied.

Adverse Effects

No serious reactions have been reported in the literature.

Possible Interactions

No interactions with other drugs or herbs have been reported in the literature. Because of the limited information available, it seems prudent not to combine *U. tomentosa* with other herbs or drugs that affect the immune system, such as cortisone-like drugs or cyclosporine.

Echinacea

Echinacea is the name of a genus of native North American plants with reddish or purplish flowers. There are nine species, but only three of them (*E. angustifolia, E. pallida, E. purpurea*) are used as botanical medicines. Gardeners may recognize echinacea as the purple coneflower.

Echinacea was used traditionally by many Native American tribes to treat snakebite and many other ailments, and settlers learned of its properties from the Indians. Most of the research on the chemistry and pharmacology of these plants has been conducted in Europe, where, until fairly recently, echinacea was a much more popular herb than in the United States.

The current enthusiasm for echinacea derives from research suggesting that it can stimulate the immune system and help fight off viral infections, such as colds or influenza. In this country, echinacea is available primarily as a tincture (alcohol-based extract) or as capsules of dried leaves and stems collected when the plant is in flower.

Active Ingredients

The three species are not interchangeable, although they may sometimes be confused with one another. Each may have a different balance of active compounds. Of course, the roots also differ from the above-ground parts of the plant, though both are utilized medicinally. The chemistry of echinacea is complex, and no single ingredient has been identified as primarily responsible for the therapeutic activity. A caffeic acid glycoside, echinacoside, makes up approximately 0.1 percent of the leaves and stems, which also contain cichoric acid. Fresh echinacea or its juice contains a volatile substance not found in the dried plant material. The roots of *E. angustifolia* contain chemicals called alkamides.

Uses

Echinacea has become extremely popular for the treatment of colds, influenza, and other respiratory tract infections. Although the herb does not seem to kill viruses directly, it is believed to stimulate or modulate the immune system, allowing the host to fight off infection. In one European study, people taking echinacea recovered from their colds four days earlier than those taking a placebo. Both the root of *E. pallida* and the above ground parts of *E. purpurea* are used in Europe for this purpose. It is usually given just at the first appearance of symptoms, rather than taken daily as a preventive.

One study of 300 people (in three groups, taking *E. purpurea*, *E. angustifolia*, or placebo) over 12 weeks was not able to demonstrate a significant advantage of the botanical medicines over placebo. The authors hypothesize that echinacea might reduce the rate of infection by 10 to 20 percent, undetectable at that sample size. The herb is given orally or by injection in Germany for other infections as well, including prostatitis and urinary tract infections.

Test-tube and animal research has shown that echinacea extracts have significant anti-inflammatory activity. When applied to the skin, the extract is almost as effective as a potent anti-inflammatory drug, indomethacin, used topically. Topically, the extracts have been used to help hasten the healing of stubborn wounds, eczema, psoriasis, and herpes simplex.

To maximize the benefit of the herb, it should be given together with a multiple vitamin. (In Australia, a formulation that includes echinacea, vitamin A, vitamin C, vitamin E, zinc, and garlic is prescribed at the first sign of viral respiratory infection.)

Preliminary studies suggest that it may be of some use in treating certain cancers. Much more research is needed on this potential application.

Dosage

When fresh-squeezed juice is used, the dose is 6 to 9 ml, or approximately 1½ teaspoons (= 7.5 ml). Other oral formulations should supply the equivalent of 900 mg of the herb daily. One study indicated that short-term use could boost cell-mediated immunity, but that repeated use over a period of weeks reduced the immune response. This interpretation of the results has been questioned, but most authorities suggest six to eight weeks as the maximum time to take echinacea preparations.

One study using the fresh juice of *E. purpurea* showed no problems for people taking it for up to 12 weeks. The herb should be stored away from light to maintain potency.

Special Precautions

Many authorities warn against using echinacea for people with autoimmune diseases, multiple sclerosis, or other serious conditions, such as tuberculosis, AIDS, or leukemia. These precautions appear to rest on theoretical grounds and are not universally accepted, but we believe it is prudent to respect them.

Adverse Reactions

Side effects have rarely been reported with the use of echinacea.

In a recent study of echinacea extracts for the prevention of colds, 18 percent of the patients taking *E. angustifolia*, 10 percent of those taking *E. purpurea*, and 11 percent of those on placebo experienced side effects.

The researchers did not specify what reactions occurred but reported that they were not serious and did not require treatment. Echinacea has an unpleasant aftertaste.

Possible Interactions

Interactions of echinacea with other medications are based on theoretical concerns. Some of the alkaloids found in echinacea are similar to plant chemicals that can be damaging to the liver. Thus, some doctors suggest that echinacea should not be used with other drugs that can have negative effects on the liver, such as Nizoral, methotrexate, Cordarone, or anabolic steroids. One reference notes that flavonoids found in *E. purpurea* affect the enzyme (CYP 3A4) responsible for metabolizing many common drugs.

This is the same enzyme affected by grapefruit, but we do not know if the effect would be clinically important. If it were, medications as varied as cyclosporine, Plendil, Procardia, Sular, Propulsid, Hismanal, Mevacor, Zocor, Tegretol, or Viagra could reach higher levels in the body. Coumadin might also be affected. Monitoring drug response is important.

Essiac Herbs

Essiac, a harmless herbal tea, was used by Canadian nurse Rene Caisse to successfully treat thousands of cancer patients from the 1920s until her death in 1978 at the age of 90. Refusing payment for her services, instead accepting only voluntary contributions, the Bracebridge, Ontario, nurse brought remissions to hundreds of documented cases, many abandoned as "hopeless" or "terminal" by orthodox medicine. She aided countless more in prolonging life and relieving pain. Caisse obtained remarkable results against a wide variety of cancers, treating persons by administering Essiac through hypodermic injection or oral ingestion.

The following benefits may result from the use of Essiac:

- Prevent build-up of excess fatty deposits in artery walls, heart, kidney tubules, and liver.
- Regulate cholesterol levels by transforming sugar and fat into energy.
- Halt diarrhea, check internal hemorrhaging, and overcome constipation.

- Counteract the detrimental effects of aluminum, lead, and mercury poisoning.
- Strengthen and tighten muscles, organs, and tissues.
- Make bones, joints, ligaments, lungs, and membranes strong and flexible, more durable, and less vulnerable to stress.
- Nourish and stimulate the brain and nervous system.
- Promote the absorption of fluids in the tissues.
- Remove toxic accumulation in the fat, lymph, bone marrow, bladder, and alimentary canal.
- Neutralize acids, absorb toxins in bowel, and help to eliminate both.
- Relieve the liver of its burden of detoxification by converting fatty toxins into water-soluble substances that can be easily eliminated through the kidneys.
- Reduce, perhaps eliminate, heavy metal deposits in tissues, especially those surrounding the joints, to relieve inflammation and stiffness.
- Improve the functions of the pancreas and spleen by increasing the effectiveness of insulin.
- Increase red cell production.
- Increase the body's ability to utilize oxygen by raising the oxygen level in tissue cells.
- Maintain the balance between potassium and sodium within the body so the fluid inside and outside each cell is regulated. In this way, cells are nourished with nutrients and are cleansed.
- Protect against toxins entering the brain.
- Protect the body against radiation and x-rays.
- Relieve pain, increase the appetite, and provide more energy with a sense of well-being.
- Speed up wound healing by regenerating the damaged area.

- Increase the production of antibodies like lymphocytes in the thymus gland, defenders of our immune system.
- Inhibit and possibly destroy benign growths and tumors.

Essiac Herbs

- Burdock Root (*Arctium lappa*)
- Sheep Sorrel (*Rumex acetosella*)
- Turkey Rhubarb Root (*Rheum palmatum*)
- Slippery Elm Bark (*Ulmus fulva*)

The herbs can be made into a tea, powdered extract, and tincture.

Garlic

Garlic is valued in many parts of the world for its pungent aroma and flavor. It is possible that garlic's biological activity and popularity in Mediterranean cuisines contribute to the healthful effects of the "Mediterranean diet."

Garlic was used in the nineteenth century for tuberculosis and into World War II for disinfecting battlefield wounds. It is frequently used in an attempt to ward off or treat the common cold. The herb is available in many forms, including fresh bulbs, oil-based extracts, dried powder, and steam-distilled extracts. To maximize the anti-cancer activity of fresh garlic in cooking, crush or mince it at least 10 minutes before heating.

Active Ingredients

Sulfur compounds give garlic its characteristic pungent aroma and probably account for some of the flavor. They also appear to be responsible for most of the medicinal properties of this herb, although the trace minerals germanium and selenium may also play a role. An inert compound, alliin, is converted to allicin once the clove is cut or crushed.

In Europe, standardized extracts of garlic are supposed to contain at least 0.45 percent allicin, a compound that breaks down into most of the active components, such as ajoene. Chemical analysis of garlic products shows that concentrations of sulfur compounds vary enormously.

Uses

Garlic is widely used for its cardiovascular benefits, although the results of two American trials on its ability to lower cholesterol were disappointing.

An analysis of 26 other studies showed that cholesterol was reduced, on the average, by approximately 10 percent.

In some studies, dangerous LDL cholesterol dropped by 16 percent while other research has shown increases in beneficial HDL with long-term use.

Although the cholesterol-lowering power of garlic appears modest, the herb is reported to reduce oxidation of LDL and seems to have other cardioprotective effects. Several garlic-derived chemicals can help slow blood clotting by keeping blood platelets from clumping together. In addition, garlic helps to break up or prevent blood clots through fibrinolytic action. Since many heart attacks and strokes are believed to be caused by spontaneous clots in blood vessels, these anticoagulant actions could be very helpful. Garlic may also lower blood pressure, but it is less effective in this respect than are medicines. It is helpful, however, in keeping blood vessels to the heart flexible in older people.

One of the most intriguing possibilities for garlic is that regular ingestion may help prevent cancer. Studies in China, comparing people in one region where garlic is commonly eaten (20 grams, or approximately seven cloves a day, on average) with those in another region where daily consumption is less than half a clove, found the garlic eaters were much less likely to suffer stomach cancer. Other studies have indicated that people who eat garlic more often seem less susceptible to stomach or colon cancer.

Animal research confirms that garlic has the potential to improve resistance to tumors, and test-tube research shows that garlic can interfere with some cancer-causing chemicals.

Adverse Effects

In rats, high doses of garlic led to weight loss and damage to the stomach lining. Humans taking garlic oil at a dose equivalent to 20 cloves daily for three months did not report problems. Most people appear to tolerate garlic well, but some individuals experience digestive distress.

People who handle garlic products occasionally develop a skin reaction on exposure (contact dermatitis). Ingesting fresh garlic and most extracts results in a characteristic breath odor. This has been linked to the active sulfur-containing compounds. Parsley is recommended as a home remedy for garlic breath.

Possible Interactions

Although there are no studies of interactions, in theory, garlic could increase the risk of bleeding in people taking anticoagulants, such as Coumadin, aspirin, Plavix, or Ticlid. There is also a possibility that this herb could interact with drugs such as DiaBeta or Glucotrol that lower blood sugar. Careful monitoring is suggested for anyone combining garlic products with such prescription drugs. Garlic appears to inhibit an enzyme called CYP 2E1. In most cases, this interference is welcome, since this enzyme can make carcinogens more dangerous. But CYP 2E1 is also involved in the metabolism of acetaminophen (Panadol, Tylenol, etc.) and a muscle relaxant called chlorzoxazone (Parafon Forte). These drugs could possibly linger longer in people who are taking or eating garlic.

Green Tea

Green tea extract is used in cancer primarily to reduce risk and enhance immune function. It contains many vitamins and minerals as well as some other important ingredients listed below.

Active Ingredients

The methylxanthine alkaloids, caffeine, theophylline, and theobromine, comprise between 1 and 5 percent of tea. These compounds have similar but not identical actions; caffeine is usually the dominant one.

Depending on the variety of tea and the way it was prepared, a cup (a proper six-ounce teacup) may contain from 10 to 50 mg of caffeine.

Low doses of caffeine may actually slow heart rate slightly while higher doses can speed heart rate or even contribute to mild rhythm abnormalities.

Green tea, like black tea, is rich in tannins. Tannic acids make up 9 to 20 percent of the leaves. Flavonoids, including apigenin, kaempferol, myricetin, and quercetin, have also been identified but at low concentrations. Some flavonoids unique to black tea are theaflavins, theasinensins, thearubigens, and theacitrins.

Another set of flavonoids have been intensively studied recently. These polyphenols (catechins) are not vitamins, but they seem to have strong antioxidant properties. Epigallocatechin-3-gallate (EGCG), in particular, has been identified as capable of protecting experimental animals from radiation damage and possibly reducing the risk of cancer.

Uses

Current interest in green tea in the United States has focused mainly on its cancer-preventive properties rather than on its flavor, which may be an acquired taste. Japanese researchers were the first to report that people living in an area where green tea was an important crop were only half or even a fifth as likely to develop cancer as those in an area that did not grow tea. There seems to be an inverse relationship between drinking tea and developing cancer of the digestive tract or urinary system. One recent epidemiological study in Japan showed that men who drank 10 or more cups of green tea daily had a significantly lower risk of lung, liver, colon, or stomach cancer.

EGCG seems to be responsible in large measure for inhibiting the growth of cancer cells and mopping up free radicals that can damage healthy cells.

It also appears to work on the heterocyclic amines that form when meat, poultry, or fish is grilled and keeps them from initiating cancerous changes.

One Chinese study suggests that green tea can counteract the cancer-promoting effects of female hormones on breast tissue. Further research on this possibility is needed. The polyphenols in green tea are thought to be responsible for its chemopreventive activity. Curcumin seems to act synergistically with green tea in preventing mutations and tumor development.

EGCG also has antibacterial and antiviral activity and stimulates the immune system to produce interleukin-1 and tumor necrosis factor. These and possibly other actions may explain the capacity of EGCG to reduce periodontitis; and this, in turn, may explain how green tea helps minimize bad breath.

Prospective trials have not shown that tea lowers blood lipids. Because tea discourages oxidation of low-density lipoprotein, however, it may help protect against atherosclerosis. Both green tea and Earl Grey counteracted platelet clumping and prevented coronary blood clots in a dog experiment, but scientists have not been able to demonstrate any anti-platelet effect in humans.

Topical application of EGCG from green tea in animal experiments stopped the development of skin cancer after exposure to a carcinogenic chemical.

Polyphenols from green tea can also protect skin from ultraviolet radiation (UV-B) damage, acting essentially as a natural sunscreen.

Dose

Approximately 2 g of tea is used with 250 ml of boiling water.

Large doses of green tea, up to nine or ten cups daily, were associated with cardiovascular benefit in the early epidemiological studies. These results have not been confirmed.

Daily use of green tea by much of the population in China and Japan suggests that no strict time limits on administration need be observed.

Special Precautions

High doses of caffeine have been linked to infertility and birth defects. Large amounts of green tea are, therefore, not recommended for pregnant women or those attempting to conceive. Caffeine is detectable in breast milk after the mother consumes a caffeine-containing beverage.

The diuretic effects of caffeine and theophylline may put a strain on kidneys with pre-existing problems. People with ulcers, heart rhythm problems, and clinical anxiety disorders should minimize their intake of caffeine.

Adverse Effects

People who drink excessive amounts of green tea may get too much caffeine. High concentrations of caffeine (hard to achieve with moderate green tea intake) can result in rapid heart rate or altered heart rhythm (PVC), excess fluid elimination, jitteriness, and insomnia.

Chronic use of caffeine can lead to symptoms of headache, sluggishness, and irritability upon withdrawal. Withdrawal has been reported in people who stop drinking as little as two or three cups of coffee daily and, therefore, might be anticipated in people who suddenly stop drinking many cups of green tea (five or six daily).

Possible Interactions

The tannins in tea can interfere with the absorption of non-heme iron (iron supplements, for example) taken at the same time. Milk added to black tea can reduce the binding capacity of tannins. (Milk is rarely, if ever, added to green tea.) Caffeine (65 mg) can increase the analgesic effects of aspirin or acetaminophen. Antibiotics, such as Cipro, Noroxin, or Penetrex, and the ulcer drug Tagamet (cimetidine), can increase the stimulant effects of caffeine. Combining tea with a medication containing theophylline or caffeine could result in too much caffeine and cause nervousness or insomnia.

Hoxsey Formula

In the early 1900s, Harry Hoxsey developed an herbal formula that he believed was effective for the treatment of cancer. It consists of two remedies: one to be used externally; the other, internally. The external mixture is said to be selectively destructive of cancerous tissue and consists of a red paste—containing antimony trisulfide, zinc chloride, and bloodroot—and a yellow powder—containing arsenic sulfide, sulfur, and talc. The internal mixture is a liquid containing licorice, red clover, burdock root, stillingia root, barberry, cascara, prickly ash bark, buckthorn bark, and potassium iodide. This mixture is considered to be cathartic/cleansing or immune-boosting. Hoxsey felt that his therapy normalized and balanced the body's chemistry makeup, allowing it to essentially create a self-healing environment in which the immune system is strengthened and tumors are caused to die. The treatment is available in Tijuana, Mexico.

Dosage

The dose of the therapy varies depending on the specific needs of each patient and whether the cancer is internal or on the skin.

The preparation is used either directly on the skin or drunk as a tonic. Patients are encouraged to *avoid* pork, vinegar, tomatoes, carbonated drinks, and alcohol, and to *use* immune stimulants, yeast tablets, vitamin C, calcium, laxatives, and antiseptic washes as well as adopt a positive mental outlook while taking the Hoxsey treatment.

Adverse Reactions

Some of the ingredients in the Hoxsey formula can cause side effects. For instance, buckthorn bark can cause nausea, vomiting, and diarrhea if taken in large quantities. Cascara can cause diarrhea. Barberry root administered to rabbits (dose unspecified) caused swelling of the kidney and cardiotoxicity.

Diarrhea can lead to dehydration and electrolyte imbalance.

Iscador

Iscador is a remedy used by European physicians. It is the trade name for the herb mistletoe. In animal experiments, Iscador has been found to kill cancer cells, stimulate the immune system, and inhibit tumor formation. Iscador is available from Waleda at 1.800.241.1030. For further information about Iscador, you may contact Health&Wellness Institute. Biological Homeopathic

Industries (BHI) has Viscum album (homeopathic mistletoe extract).

Milk Thistle (Silybum marianum)

This herb is grown in varied places. You may find it along roadsides and grown wild in different climates. The seeds of the dried flower are used. In cancer, this herb is primarily used in chemotherapy support. It enhances liver detoxification and supports the growth of healthy liver cells.

Uses

Milk thistle has a history of being used for hundreds of years. It was prescribed in liver and gallbladder conditions often. It was used in the treatment of jaundice. This herb is an all-around safe and effective medicine.

Milk thistle contains a bioflavonoid known as silymarin. Silymarin is made up of three constituents: silibinin, silidianin, and silicristin. The action of silibinin is responsible for medicinal benefits of silymarin. Milk thistle protects liver cells against toxins and is known to cause the healthy growth of new liver cells.

Dosage

Milk thistle is relatively safe and devoid of any side effects. In liver disease, it is recommended 400-1,000 mg of milk thistle be given. If you prefer to use it in the form of food, 12-15 grams of seeds can be ground. However, this by no means will have a therapeutic effect on the liver.

Adverse Reactions

Milk thistle is free from any side effects and can be used in a wide range of health conditions. Some may notice a mild laxative effect with using this herb.

Contraindications and Possible Interactions

None currently known.

Mushroom Extract

Shiitake and Maitake mushroom extracts and isolates have been used in a variety of cancers. Maitake mushroom extracts demonstrate more powerful antitumor properties. Maitake has inhibiting effects on carcinogenesis (development of cancer) and metastasis (the spread of cancer). Shiitake is also used in cancer, but it is not as strong of an anticancer variety.

Pau d'Arco (*Tabebuia impetiginosa*; *Tabebuia avellanedae*)

Pau d'arco, known as lapacho colorado in Argentina and Paraguay and as ipe roxo in Brazil, is a good example of the lure of the exotic. This South American native has been used medicinally by several indigenous groups.

There are several species of *Tabebuia*, and most appear to be broad-leaved evergreen trees with very hard wood that resists decay. It may be difficult to determine precisely which species is being sold as pau d'arco tea.

Pau d'arco has a reputation for having been used by the Incas, although it is not native to the high Andes.

Uses

It is said to be useful against cancer, diabetes, rheumatism, and ulcers, as well as several other ailments. The part of the tree used is the inner bark, and the preparation made from it is sometimes termed *taheebo*.

Pau d'arco, or taheebo, contains a number of quinone compounds, including the naphthoquinone lapachol and the anthraquinone tabebuin. These and related compounds are assumed to be the active ingredients.

Lapachol has antibacterial activity, and a related compound fights off fungus and yeast. Lapachol has demonstrated activity against malaria, a property that would certainly be useful for people in the areas where *Tabebuia* species grow wild.

Test-tube and animal research in the 1950s and 1960s indicated that taheebo extract and lapachol could slow the growth of certain tumors.

In human trials, it was difficult to attain therapeutically active levels of lapachol with oral administration, and when levels did get high enough, most people suffered serious adverse effects, such as nausea and vomiting.

Taheebo extract has anti-inflammatory activity, at least in rats. Researchers have also found that it helps animals resist ulcers. In laboratory studies on human blood cells, lapachol had immunosuppressant effects at higher doses and immunostimulant activity at low doses.

Dosage

Standard dose has not been determined.

Contraindications

Pregnant women should not take taheebo internally because there is no evidence of its safety, and it can provoke adverse reactions.

Pau d'arco should be discontinued before surgery because of the danger of excessive bleeding. Studies of pau d'arco in humans have noted reactions, such as severe nausea, vomiting, diarrhea, dizziness, anemia, and bleeding. Administering vitamin K will stop the bleeding.

The fact that taheebo causes vitamin K-reversible bleeding strongly suggests that it would interact with anticoagulants, such as Coumadin, to increase the danger of hemorrhage.

Pectin

Pectin has demonstrated some useful effects in stopping the spread of cancer in animal studies. It is a fiber derived from citrus and tolerated well by the body. Pectin is known to increase immune activity against cancer cells. It comes as a powder and can be taken in juice or water. For cancers that have spread to other sites, it is important to include this in the cancer treatment regimen.

Traditional Chinese Herbs

There are many traditional Chinese herbs that are currently used in the treatment of cancer:

Fu Zhen therapy

Used in hospitals in China for the treatment of cancer. This therapy increases the activity of nonspecific immune cells. The following herbs are used in this treatment: ginseng, ligustrum, astragalus, codonopsis, astracylodes, and ganoderma. The aim of therapy is to restore energy, enhance digestion, and strengthen the immune system.

Liu Wei Di Huang

Used primarily in lung cancer. It is also known as the Six Flavor Tea. This Chinese formulation is said to have antitumor effects.

Jian Pi Yi Qi Li Shui (Polyporus umbellatus)

This herb is used to reduce the risk of injury to the kidneys while undergoing chemotherapy. It also exhibits antitumor effects by stimulating immune activity around tumor sites.

PC SPES

Used as an herbal cancer treatment protocol for the prostate. It is also demonstrating some benefits in other forms of cancer including sarcoma and breast cancer, although this formulation is not used primarily in these cancers. PC SPES is a Chinese herbal formulation and demonstrates the following activities:

1. Immune-stimulating

2. Anti-tumor

3. Anti-viral

4. Anti-inflammatory

5. Decreased bioavailability of testosterone

The following herbs are in the formulation:

- Isatis indigotica (da qing ye)
- Glycyrrhiza glabra and Gycyrrhiza uralensis (gan cao) also known as licorice root
- Panax ginseng (san qi)
- Ganoderma lucidum (ling zhi)
- Scutellaria baicalensis (huang qin)
- Dendranthema (chrysanthemum)
- Rabdosia rebescens
- Saw palmetto (serenoa repens)

Each of these herbs works together in enhancing immune action, inducing apoptosis (programmed cancer cell death), working against the tumor, increasing NK cell activity, modulating hormonal balance, and maintaining homeostasis (system balance).

For further information on PC SPES contact:

Dr. John A. Catanzaro
Health&Wellness Institute
5603 230th St. S.W.
Mountlake Terrace, Wa 98043
425.697.6112

The Best Options for Diagnosing and Treating Prostate Cancer by James Lewis Jr., Ph.D. ISBN 1-883257-04-2

The Herbal Remedy for Prostate Cancer by James Lewis Jr., Ph.D. ISBN 1-883257-02-6

Other traditional Chinese herbs can be referenced in the book *Cancer and Natural Medicine.** This book is an excellent resource for identifying potentially useful herbs in cancer treatment.

---

* Written by John Boik. Oregon Medical Press. ISBN 0-9648280-0-6.

Conventional Cancer Treatments

Both conventional and alternative medicine have much to offer in cancer treatment.

In conventional treatment, it is common to use chemotherapy, surgery, radiation, and biological therapy. These therapies may be used in combination, depending upon the type of cancer. In this section, we will briefly discuss chemotherapy and radiotherapy, which is also called radiation therapy.

Chemotherapy

There are many forms of chemotherapy with varied results. Not all regimens are the same. It is always prudent to implement integrative treatment to combat the negative effects of chemotherapy. You may not be settled with chemotherapy or you may be unsure as to whether it is right for you. This is why it is vital to research and get the expertise advice from your oncologist and alternative health care physician before making a decision.

How Does Chemotherapy Work?

Normal cells grow and die in a controlled way. When cancer occurs, cells in the body that are not normal keep dividing and forming more cells without control. Anticancer drugs destroy cancer cells by stopping them from growing or multiplying. Healthy cells can also be harmed, especially those that divide quickly. Harm to healthy cells is what causes side effects. These cells usually repair themselves after chemotherapy.

What Can Chemotherapy Do?

Depending on the type of cancer and how advanced it is, chemotherapy can be used for different goals:

- To cure the cancer. Cancer is considered cured when the patient remains free of evidence of cancer cells.
- To control the cancer. This is done by keeping the cancer from spreading, slowing the cancer's growth, and killing cancer cells that may have spread to other parts of the body from the original tumor.
- To relieve symptoms that the cancer may cause. Relieving symptoms, such as pain, can help patients live more comfortably.

Is Chemotherapy Used with Other Treatments?

Sometimes chemotherapy is the only treatment a patient receives. More often, however, chemotherapy is used in addition to surgery, and/or biological therapy to:

- Shrink a tumor before surgery or radiation therapy. This is called neo-adjuvant therapy.
- Help destroy any cancer cells that may remain after surgery and/or radiation therapy. This is called adjuvant chemotherapy.
- Make radiation therapy and biological therapy work better.

- Help destroy cancer if it recurs or has spread to other parts of the body from the original tumor.

Which Drugs Are Given?

Some chemotherapy drugs are used for many different types of cancer, while others might be used for just one or two types of cancer.

Your doctor recommends a treatment plan based on:

- What kind of cancer you have.
- What part of the body the cancer is found in.
- The effect of cancer on your normal body functions.
- Your general health.

What About Clinical Trials?

Clinical trials test many types of treatments, such as new drugs, new approaches to surgery or radiation therapy, new combinations of treatments, or new methods such as gene therapy. The goal of this research is to find better ways to treat cancer and help cancer patients. There are different types of clinical trials: Phase I, Phase II, and Phase III trials. Each is one of the final stages of a long and careful cancer research process. If your doctor does not suggest you take part in a clinical trial, you may want to ask about clinical trials as a treatment choice for you.

Possible benefits of clinical trials include:

- Clinical trials offer high-quality cancer care.
- If a new treatment approach is proven to work and you are taking it, you may be among the first to benefit.
- By looking at the pros and cons of clinical trials and other treatment choices, you are taking an active role in a decision that affects your life.
- You have the chance to help others and improve cancer treatment.

Possible drawbacks:

- New treatments under study are not always better than, or even as good as, standard treatment.
- Even if a new treatment has benefits, it may not work for you.
- In a study, if you are randomly assigned to have standard treatment instead of the new treatment being tested, it may not be as effective as the new approach.
- Health insurance and managed care providers do not always cover all patient care costs in a study.

Before deciding to join a clinical trial, you will want to ask important questions such as: What are the possible short- and long-term risks, side effects, and benefits to me? How could the study affect my daily life? Will I have to pay for any treatment, tests, or other charges?

Ask Your Doctor

About Chemotherapy

- Why do I need chemotherapy?
- What are the benefits of chemotherapy?
- What are the risks of chemotherapy?
- Are there any other possible treatment methods for my type of cancer?
- What is the standard care for my type of cancer?
- Are there any clinical trials for my type of cancer?

About Your Treatment

- How many treatments will I be given?
- What drug or drugs will I be taking?
- How will the drugs be given?
- Where will I get my treatment?
- How long will each treatment last?

About Side Effects

- What are the possible side effects of the chemotherapy?
- When are side effects likely to occur?
- What side effects are more likely to be related to my type of cancer?
- Are there any side effects that I should report right away?
- What can I do to relieve the side effects?

About Contacting Medical Staff

- How do I contact a health professional after hours, and when should I call?

Hints for Talking with Your Doctor

These tips might help you keep track of the information you learn during visits with your doctor:

- Bring a friend or family member to sit with you while you talk with your doctor. This person can help you understand what your doctor says during your visit and help refresh your memory afterward.
- Ask your doctor for printed information that is available on your cancer and treatment.
- You, or the person who goes with you, may want to take notes during your appointment.
- Ask your doctor to slow down when you need more time to write.

You may want to ask if you can use a tape recorder during your visit. Take notes from the tape after the visit is finished. That way, you can review your conversation later as many times as you wish.

How Often and For How Long Will I Get Chemotherapy?

How often and how long you get chemotherapy depends on:

- The kind of cancer you have.
- The goals of the treatment.
- The drugs that are used.
- How your body responds to them.

You may get treatment every day, every week, or every month. Chemotherapy is often given in cycles that include treatment periods alternated with rest periods. Rest periods give your body a chance to build healthy new cells and regain its strength. Ask your health care provider to tell you how long and how often you may expect to get treatment.

Sticking with your treatment schedule is very important for the drugs to work right. Schedules may need to be changed for holidays and other reasons. If you miss a treatment session or skip a dose of the drug, contact your doctor.

Sometimes, your doctor may need to delay a treatment based on the results of certain blood tests. Your doctor will let you know what to do during this time and when to start your treatment again.

How Is Chemotherapy Given?

Chemotherapy can be given in several different ways: intravenously (through a vein), by mouth, through an injection (shot), or applied on the skin.

By Vein (intravenous, or IV, treatment).

Chemotherapy is most often given intravenously (IV) through a vein. Usually, a thin needle is inserted into a vein on the hand or lower arm at the beginning of each treatment session and is removed at the end of the session. If you feel a coolness, burning, or other unusual sensation in the area of the needle stick when the IV is started, tell your doctor or nurse. Also report any pain, burning, skin redness, swelling, or discomfort that occurs during or after an IV treatment.

Chemotherapy can also be delivered by IV through catheters, ports, and pumps.

A catheter is a soft, thin, flexible tube that is placed in a large vein in the body and remains there as long as it is needed.

Patients who need to have many IV treatments often have a catheter, so a needle does not have to be used each time. Drugs can be given and blood samples can be drawn through this catheter. Sometimes, the catheter is attached to a small, round, plastic or metal disc placed under the skin. The port can be used for as long as it is needed.

A pump, which is used to control how fast the drug goes into a catheter or port, is sometimes used. There are two types of pumps. An external pump remains outside the body. Most are portable; they allow a person to move around while the pump is being used. An internal pump is placed inside the body during surgery, usually right under the skin. Pumps contain a small storage area for the drug and allow people to go about their normal activities.

Catheters, ports, and pumps cause no pain if they are properly placed and cared for, although a person is aware they are there.

By Mouth (orally).

The drug is given in pill, capsule, or liquid form. You swallow the drug, just as you do many other medicines.

By Injection.

A needle and syringe are used to give the drug in one of several ways:

- Intramuscular or IM (into a muscle).
- Subcutaneous or SQ or SC (under the skin).
- Intralesion or IL (directly into a cancerous area in the skin).

Topically.

The drug is applied on the surface of the skin.

How Will I Feel During Chemotherapy?

Most people receiving chemotherapy find that they tire easily, but many feel well enough to continue to lead active lives. Each person and treatment is different, so it is not always possible to tell exactly how you will react. Your general state of health, the type and extent of cancer you have, and the kind of drugs you are receiving can all affect how well you feel.

You may want to have someone available to drive you to and from treatment if, for example, you are taking medicine for nausea or vomiting that could make you tired. You may also feel especially tired from the chemotherapy as early as one day after a treatment and for several days afterwards. It may help to schedule your treatment when you can take off the day of and the day after your treatment. If you have young children, you may want to schedule the treatment when you have someone to help at home the day of and at least the day after your treatment. Ask your doctor when your greatest fatigue or other side effects are likely to occur.

Most people can continue working while receiving chemotherapy. However, you may need to change your work schedule for a while if your chemotherapy makes you feel very tired or have other side effects. Talk with your employer about your needs and wishes. You may be able to agree on a part-time schedule, find an area for a short nap during the day, or perhaps you can do some of your work at home.

Under federal and state laws, some employers may be required to let you work a flexible schedule to meet your treatment needs. To find out about your on-the-job protections, check with a social worker or your congressional or state representative.

Can I Take Other Medicines While I Am Getting Chemotherapy?

Some medicines may interfere or react with the effects of your chemotherapy. Give your doctor a list of all the medicines you take before you start treatment. Include:

- the name of each drug.
- the dosage.
- the reason you take it.
- how often you take it.

How Will I Know If My Chemotherapy Is Working?

Your doctor and nurse will use several ways to see how well your treatments are working. You may have physical exams and tests often. Always feel free to ask your doctor about the test results and what they show about your progress.

Tests and exams can tell a lot about how chemotherapy is working; however, side effects tell very little. Sometimes, people think that if they have no side effects, the drugs are not working; or if they do have side effects, the drugs are working well. But side effects vary so much from person to person and from drug to drug that they are not a sign of whether the treatment is working or not.

Side Effects Encountered During Chemotherapy

What Causes Side Effects?

Because cancer cells may grow and divide more rapidly than normal cells, many anticancer drugs are made to kill growing cells. But certain normal, healthy cells also multiply quickly, and chemotherapy can affect these cells too. This damage to normal cells causes side effects. The fast-growing, normal cells most likely to be affected are blood cells forming in the bone and cells in the digestive tract (mouth, stomach, intestines, esophagus), reproductive system (sexual organs), and hair follicles. Some anticancer drugs may affect cells of vital organs, such as the heart, kidney, bladder, lungs, and nervous system.

You may have none of these side effects or just a few. The kinds of side effects you have, and how severe they are, depend on the type and dose of chemotherapy you get and how your body reacts to it. Before starting chemotherapy, your doctor will discuss the side effects that you are most likely to get with the drugs you will be receiving. Before starting the treatment, you will be asked to sign a consent form. You should be given all the facts about treatment, including the drugs you will be given and their side effects, before you sign the consent form.

How Long Do Side Effects Last?

Normal cells usually recover when chemotherapy is over, so most side effects gradually go away after treatment ends and the healthy cells have a chance to grow normally. The time it takes to get over side effects depends on many things, including your overall health and the kind of chemotherapy you have been taking.

On some occasions, chemotherapy can cause permanent changes or damage to the heart, lungs, nerves, kidneys, reproductive or other organs. And certain types of chemotherapy may have delayed effects, such as a second cancer that shows up many years later. Ask your doctor about the chances of any serious, long-term effects that can result from the treatment you are receiving (but remember to balance your concerns with the immediate threat of your cancer).

Great progress has been made in preventing and treating some of chemotherapy's common, as well as rare, serious side effects. Many new drugs and treatment methods destroy cancer more effectively while doing less harm to the body's healthy cells.

The side effects of chemotherapy can be unpleasant, but they must be measured against the treatment's ability to destroy cancer. Medicines can help prevent some side effects, such as nausea. Sometimes, people receiving chemotherapy become discouraged about the length of time their treatment is taking or the side effects they are having. If that happens to you, talk to your doctor or nurse. They may be able to suggest ways to make side effects easier to deal with or reduce them.

It is essential to consider integrating your therapy with proper nutritional replacement. In many cases, the body is deprived of vital nutrients and minerals that the chemotherapy depletes. IV nutritional replacement is recommended. Some of the common side effects can improve, if not be abated, by nutritional support therapy.

Below, you will find suggestions for dealing with some of the more common side effects of chemotherapy.

Fatigue

Fatigue, feeling tired and lacking energy, is the most common symptom reported by cancer patients. The exact cause is not always known. It can be due to your disease, chemotherapy, radiation, surgery, low blood counts, lack of sleep, pain, stress, or poor appetite, along with many other factors.

Fatigue from cancer feels different from fatigue of everyday life. Fatigue caused by chemotherapy can appear suddenly. Patients with cancer have described it as a total lack of energy and have used words such as "worn out," "drained," and "wiped out" to describe their fatigue. And rest does not always relieve it. Not everyone feels the same kind of fatigue. You may not feel tired while someone else does, or your fatigue may not last as long as someone else's does. It can last days, weeks, or months. But severe fatigue does go away gradually as the tumor responds to treatment.

How can I cope with fatigue?

- Plan your day so that you have time to rest.
- Take short naps or breaks, rather than one long rest period.
- Save your energy for the most important things.
- Try easier or shorter versions of activities you enjoy.
- Take short walks or do light exercise if possible. You may find this helps with fatigue.
- Talk to your health care provider about ways to save your energy and treat your fatigue.
- Eat as well as you can and drink plenty of fluids. Eat small amounts at a time if it is helpful.
- Join a support group. Sharing your feelings with others can ease the burden of fatigue. You can learn how others deal with their fatigue. Your health care

provider can put you in touch with a support group in your area.

- Limit the amount of caffeine and alcohol you drink.
- Allow others to do some things for you that you usually do.
- Keep a diary of how you feel each day. This will help you plan your daily activities.
- Report any changes in energy level to your doctor or nurse.

Nausea and Vomiting

Many patients fear that they will have nausea and vomiting while receiving chemotherapy. But new drugs have made these side effects far less common and, when they do occur, much less severe. Antinausea drugs can prevent or lessen nausea and vomiting in most patients. Different drugs work for different people, and you may need more than one drug to get relief. Do not give up. Continue to work with your doctor and nurse to find the drug or drugs that work best for you. Also, be sure to tell your doctor or nurse if you are very nauseated or have vomited for more than a day, or if your vomiting is so bad that you cannot keep liquids down.

What can I do if I have nausea and vomiting?

- Drink liquids at least an hour before or after mealtime, instead of with your meals. Drink frequently and drink small amounts.
- Eat and drink slowly.
- Eat small meals throughout the day, instead of one, two, or three large meals.
- Eat foods cold or at room temperature so you won't be bothered by strong smells.
- Chew your food well for easier digestion.
- If nausea is a problem in the morning, try eating dry foods like cereal, toast, or crackers before getting up.

(Do not try this if you have mouth or throat sores, or are troubled by a lack of saliva.)

- Drink cool, clear, unsweetened fruit juices, such as apple or grape juice (or light-colored sodas, such as ginger ale, that have lost their fizz and do not have caffeine).
- Suck on mints or tart candies. (Do not use tart candies if you have mouth or throat sores.)
- Prepare and freeze meals in advance for days when you do not feel like cooking.
- Wear loose-fitting clothes.
- Breathe deeply and slowly when you feel nauseated.
- Distract yourself by chatting with friends or family members, listening to music, or watching a movie or TV show.
- Use relaxation techniques.
- Try to avoid odors that bother you, such as cooking smells, smoke, or perfume.
- Avoid sweet, fried, or fatty foods.
- Rest, but do not lie flat for at least 2 hours, after you finish a meal.
- Avoid eating for at least a few hours before treatment if nausea usually occurs during chemotherapy.
- Eat a light meal before treatment.

Pain

Chemotherapy drugs can cause some side effects that are painful. The drugs can damage nerves, leading to burning, numbness, tingling, or shooting pain, most often in the fingers or toes. Some drugs can also cause mouth sores, headaches, muscle pains, and stomach pains.

Not everyone with cancer or who receives chemotherapy experiences pain from the disease or its treatment. But if you do, it can be relieved. The first step to take is to talk with your doctor, nurse, and pharmacist about your pain. They need to know as many details about your pain as possible. You may want to describe your pain to your family and friends. They can help you talk to your caregivers about your pain, especially if you are too tired or in too much pain to talk to them yourself.

You need to tell your doctor, nurse, pharmacist, and family or friends:

- where you feel pain.
- what it feels like — sharp, dull, throbbing, steady.
- how strong the pain feels.
- how long it lasts.
- what eases the pain; what makes the pain worse.
- what medicines you are taking for the pain, and how much relief you get from them.

Using a pain scale is helpful in describing how much pain you are feeling. Try to assign a number from 0 to 10 to your pain level. If you have no pain, use a 0. As the numbers get higher, they stand for pain that is getting worse. A 10 means the pain is as bad as it can be. You may wish to use your own pain scale, using numbers from 0 to 5 or even 0 to 100. Be sure to let others know what pain scale you are using, and use the same scale each time. For example, "My pain is 7 on a scale of 0 to 10."

The goal of pain control is to prevent pain that can be prevented, and treat the pain that can't. To do this:

- If you have persistent or chronic pain, take your pain medicine on a regular schedule (by the clock).
- Do not skip doses of your scheduled pain medicine. If you wait to take pain medicine until you feel pain, it is harder to control.
- Try using relaxation exercises at the same time you take medicine for the pain. This may help to lessen tension, reduce anxiety, and manage pain.
- Some people with chronic or persistent pain that is usually controlled by medicine can have

breakthrough pain. This occurs when moderate to severe pain "breaks through" or is felt for a short time. If you experience this pain, use a short-acting medicine ordered by your doctor. Don't wait for the pain to get worse. If you do, it may be harder to control.

There are many different medicines and methods available to control cancer pain. You should expect your doctor to seek all the information and resources necessary to make you as comfortable as possible. If you are in pain and your doctor has no further suggestions, ask to see a pain specialist or have your doctor consult with a pain specialist. A pain specialist may be an oncologist, anesthesiologist, neurologist, neurosurgeon, other doctor, nurse, or pharmacist.

Hair Loss

Hair loss is a common side effect of chemotherapy, but not all drugs cause hair loss. Your doctor can tell you if hair loss might occur with the drug or drugs you are taking. When hair loss does occur, the hair may become thinner or fall out entirely. Hair loss can occur on all parts of the body, including the head, face, arms and legs, underarms, and pubic area. The hair usually grows back after the treatments are over. Some people even start to get their hair back while they are still having treatments. Sometimes, hair may grow back a different color or texture.

Hair loss does not always happen right away. It may begin several weeks after the first treatment or after a few treatments. Many people say their head becomes sensitive before losing hair. Hair may fall out gradually or in clumps. Any hair that is still growing may become dull and dry.

How can I care for my scalp and hair during chemotherapy?

- Use a mild shampoo.
- Use a soft hairbrush.
- Use low heat when drying your hair.

- Have your hair cut short. A shorter style will make your hair look thicker and fuller. It also will make hair loss easier to manage if it occurs.
- Use a sunscreen, sunblock, hat, or scarf to protect your scalp from the sun if you lose hair on your head.
- Avoid brush rollers to set your hair.
- Avoid dying, perming, or relaxing your hair.

Some people who lose all or most of their hair choose to wear turbans, scarves, caps, wigs, or hair pieces. Others leave their head uncovered. Still others switch back and forth, depending on whether they are in public or at home with friends and family members. There are no "right" or "wrong" choices; do whatever feels comfortable for you.

If you choose to cover your head:

- Get your wig or hairpiece before you lose a lot of hair. That way, you can match your current hair style and color. You may be able to buy a wig or hairpiece at a specialty shop just for cancer patients. Someone may even come to your home to help you. You also can buy a wig or hair piece through a catalog or by phone.
- You may also consider borrowing a wig or hairpiece, rather than buying one. Check with the nurse or social work department at your hospital about resources for free wigs in your community.
- Take your wig to your hairdresser or the shop where it was purchased for styling and cutting to frame your face.
- Some health insurance policies cover the cost of a hairpiece needed because of cancer treatment. It is also a tax-deductible expense. Be sure to check your policy and ask your doctor for a "prescription."

Losing hair from your head, face, or body can be hard to accept. Feeling angry or depressed is common and perfectly all right. At the same time, keep in mind that it is a temporary side effect.

Talking about your feelings can help. If possible, share your thoughts with someone who has had a similar experience.

Anemia

Chemotherapy can reduce the bone marrow's ability to make red blood cells, which carry oxygen to all parts of your body. When there are too few red blood cells, body tissues do not get enough oxygen to do their work. This condition is called anemia. Anemia can make you feel short of breath, very weak, and tired.

Call your doctor if you have any of these symptoms:

- Fatigue (feeling very weak and tired).
- Dizziness or feeling faint.
- Shortness of breath.
- Feeling as if your heart is "pounding" or beating very fast.

Your doctor will check you often during your treatment. She or he may also prescribe a medicine, such as *epigen* or *erythropoietin*, that can boost the growth of your red blood cells. Discuss this with your doctor if you become anemic often. If your red blood cell count falls too low, you may need a blood transfusion or a medicine called erythropoietin to raise the number of red blood cells in your body.

Things you can do if you are anemic:

- Get plenty of rest. Sleep more at night and take naps during the day if you can.
- Limit your activities. Do only the things that are essential or most important to you.
- Ask for help when you need it. Ask family and friends to pitch in with things like child care, shopping, housework, or driving.
- Eat a well-balanced diet.
- When sitting, get up slowly. When lying down, sit first, and then stand. This will help prevent dizziness.

Reduction in white blood cells (WBCs) is also common in chemotherapy treatment. In these cases, great care must be taken to stay away from people with colds, the flu, or any other possible threatening infection. In cases where WBCs are low, a biological drug called *Neupogen* (Colony Stimulating Factor) is given to increase the number of white blood cells.

Central Nervous System Problems

Chemotherapy can interfere with certain functions in your central nervous system (brain), causing tiredness, confusion, and depression. These feelings will go away, once the chemotherapy dose is lowered or you finish chemotherapy. Call your doctor if these symptoms occur.

Infection

Chemotherapy can make you more likely to get infections. This happens because most anticancer drugs affect the bone marrow, making it harder to make WBCs, the cells that fight many types of infections. Your doctor will check your blood cell count often while you are getting chemotherapy. As previously mentioned, Neupogen (Colony Stimulating Factor) is used to raise WBC level to reduce the risk of infection.

Most infections come from bacteria normally found on your skin and in your mouth, intestines, and genital tract. Sometimes, the cause of an infection may not be known. Even if you take extra care, you still may get an infection. But there are some things you can do.

How can I help prevent infections?

- Wash your hands often during the day. Be sure to wash them before you eat, after you use the bathroom, and after touching animals.
- Clean your rectal area gently but thoroughly after each bowel movement. Ask your doctor or nurse for advice if the area becomes irritated or if you have hemorrhoids. Also, check with your doctor before using enemas or suppositories.

- Stay away from people who have illnesses you can catch, such as a cold, the flu, measles, or chicken pox.
- Try to avoid crowds. For example, go shopping or to the movies when the stores or theaters are least likely to be busy.
- Stay away from children who recently have received "live virus" vaccines, such as chicken pox and oral polio, since they may be contagious to people with a low blood cell count. Call your doctor or local health department if you have any questions.
- Do not cut or tear the cuticles of your nails.
- Be careful not to cut or nick yourself when using scissors, needles, or knives.
- Use an electric shaver instead of a razor to prevent breaks or cuts in your skin.
- Maintain good mouth care.
- Do not squeeze or scratch pimples.
- Take a warm (not hot) bath, shower, or sponge bath every day. Pat your skin dry using a light touch. Do not rub too hard.
- Use lotion or oil to soften and heal your skin if it becomes dry and cracked.
- Clean cuts and scrapes right away and daily with warm water, soap, and an antiseptic until healed.
- Avoid contact with animal litterboxes and waste, bird cages, and fish tanks.
- Avoid standing water, such as bird baths, flower vases, or humidifiers.
- Wear protective gloves when gardening or cleaning up after others, especially small children.
- Do not get any immunizations, such as flu or pneumonia shots, without checking with your doctor first.
- Do not eat raw fish, seafood, meat, or eggs.

These recommendations can improve your quality of life while on chemotherapy and facilitate the healing process. The above recommendations are consistent with the National Cancer Institute.

Radiotherapy

There are many forms of radiotherapy with varied results. Not all regimens are the same. It is always prudent to implement integrative treatment to combat the negative effects of radiation. You may not be settled with radiotherapy or you may be unsure as to whether it is right for you. This is why it is vital to research and get the expertise advice from your oncologist and alternative health care physician before making a decision.

Radiotherapy, also called radiation therapy, is the treatment of cancer and other diseases with ionizing radiation. Ionizing radiation deposits energy that injures or destroys cells in the area being treated (the "target tissue") by damaging their genetic material, making it impossible for these cells to continue to grow. Although radiation damages both cancer cells and normal cells, the latter are able to repair themselves and function properly. Radiotherapy may be used to treat localized solid tumors, such as cancers of the skin, tongue, larynx, brain, breast, or uterine cervix. It can also be used to treat leukemia (cancer of the blood-forming cells) and lymphoma (cancer of the lymphatic system).

One type of radiation therapy commonly used involves photons or "packets" of energy. X-rays were the first form of photon radiation to be used to treat cancer. Depending on the amount of energy they possess, the rays can be used to destroy cancer cells on the surface of or deeper in the body. The higher the energy of the x-ray beam, the deeper the x-rays can go into the target tissue. Linear accelerators and betatrons are machines that produce x-rays of increasingly greater energy. The use of machines to focus radiation (such as x-rays) on a cancer site is called external beam radiotherapy.

Gamma rays are another form of photons used in radiotherapy. Gamma rays are produced spontaneously as certain elements (such as radium, uranium, and cobalt 60) and release radiation as they decompose or decay. Each element decays at a specific rate and gives off energy in the form of gamma rays and other particles. X-rays and gamma rays have the same effect on cancer cells.

Another technique for delivering radiation to cancer cells is to place radioactive implants directly in a tumor or body cavity. This is called internal radiotherapy. (Brachytherapy, interstitial irradiation, and intracavitary irradiation are types of internal radiotherapy.) In this treatment, the radiation dose is concentrated in a small area, and the patient stays in the hospital for a few days. Internal radiotherapy is frequently used for cancers of the tongue, uterus, and cervix.

Several new approaches to radiation therapy are being evaluated to determine their effectiveness in treating cancer. One such technique is intraoperative irradiation, in which a large dose of external radiation is directed at the tumor and surrounding tissue during surgery.

Another investigational approach is particle beam radiation therapy. This type of therapy differs from photon radiotherapy in that it involves the use of fast-moving subatomic particles to treat localized cancers. A very sophisticated machine is needed to produce and accelerate the particles required for this procedure. Some particles (neutrons, pions, and heavy ions) deposit more energy along the path they take through tissue than do x-rays or gamma rays, thus causing more damage to the cells they hit. This type of radiation is often referred to as high linear energy transfer (high LET) radiation.

Scientists also are looking for ways to increase the effectiveness of radiation therapy. Two types of investigational drugs are being studied for their effect on cells undergoing radiation. Radiosensitizers make the tumor cells more likely to be damaged, and radioprotectors protect normal tissues from the effects of radiation. Hyperthermia, the use of heat, is also being studied for its effectiveness in sensitizing tissue to radiation.

Other recent radiotherapy research has focused on the use of radiolabeled antibodies to deliver doses of radiation directly to the cancer site (radioimmunotherapy). Antibodies are highly specific proteins that are made by the body in response to the presence of antigens (substances recognized as foreign by the immune system). Some tumor cells contain specific antigens that trigger the production of tumor-specific antibodies. Large quantities of these antibodies can be made in the laboratory and attached to radioactive substances (a process known as radiolabeling). Once injected into the body, the antibodies actively seek out the cancer cells, which are destroyed by the cell-killing (cytotoxic) action of the radiation. This approach can minimize the risk of radiation damage to healthy cells. The success of this technique will depend upon both the identification of appropriate radioactive substances and determination of the safe and effective dose of radiation that can be delivered in this way.

Radiation therapy may be used alone or in combination with chemotherapy or surgery. Like all forms of cancer treatment, radiation therapy can have side effects. Possible side effects of treatment with radiation include temporary or permanent loss of hair in the area being treated, skin irritation, temporary change in skin color in the treated area, and tiredness. Other side effects are largely dependent on the area of the body that is treated.

What Are the Side Effects of Treatment?

External radiation therapy does not cause your body to become radioactive. There is no need to avoid being with other people because you are undergoing treatment. Even hugging, kissing, or having sexual relations with others poses no risk of radiation exposure.

Most side effects of radiation therapy are related to the area that is being treated. Many patients have no side effects at all. Your doctor and nurse will tell you about the possible side effects you might expect and how you should deal with them. You should contact your doctor or nurse if you have any unusual symptoms during your treatment, such as coughing, sweating, fever, or pain.

The side effects of radiation therapy, although unpleasant, are usually not serious and can be controlled with medication or diet. They usually go away within a few weeks after treatment ends, although some side effects can last longer. Always check with your doctor or nurse about how you should deal with side effects.

Throughout your treatment, your doctor will regularly check on the effects of the treatment. You may not be aware of changes in the cancer, but you probably will notice decreases in pain, bleeding, or other discomfort. You may continue to notice further improvement after your treatment is completed.

Your doctor may recommend periodic tests and physical exams to be sure that the radiation is causing as little damage to normal cells as possible. Depending on the area being treated, you may have routine blood tests to check the levels of red blood cells, white blood cells, and platelets because radiation treatment can cause decreases in the levels of different blood cells.

What Can I Do To Take Care of Myself During Therapy?

Each patient's body responds to radiation therapy in its own way. That's why your doctor must plan and sometimes adjust your treatment. In addition, your doctor or nurse will give you suggestions for caring for yourself at home that are specific for your treatment and the possible side effects.

Nearly all cancer patients receiving radiation therapy need to take special care of themselves to protect their health and to help the treatment succeed. Some guidelines to remember are given on the following pages:

- Before starting treatment, be sure your doctor knows about any medicines you are taking and if you have any allergies. Do not start taking any medicine (whether prescription or over-the-counter) during your radiation therapy without first telling your doctor or nurse.

- Fatigue is common during radiation therapy. Your body will use a lot of extra energy over the course of your treatment, and you may feel very tired.

- Be sure to get plenty of rest and sleep as often as you feel the need. It's common for fatigue to last for 4 to 6 weeks after your treatment has been completed.

- Good nutrition is very important. Try to eat a balanced diet that will prevent weight loss.

- Check with your doctor who specializes in natural medicine before taking nutritional and herbal preparations during treatment.

- Avoid wearing tight clothes, such as girdles or close-fitting collars, over the treatment area.

- Wear loose, soft cotton clothing over the treated area.

- Do not wear starched or stiff clothing over the treated area.

- Be extra kind to your skin in the treatment area.

- Ask your doctor or nurse if you may use soaps, lotions, deodorants, sun blocks, medicines, perfumes, cosmetics, talcum powder, or other substances in the treated area.

- Do not scratch, rub, or scrub treated skin.

- Do not use adhesive tape on treated skin. If bandaging is necessary, use paper tape and apply it outside the treatment area. Your nurse can help you place dressings so that you can avoid irritating the treated area.

- Do not apply heat or cold (heating pad, ice pack, etc.) to the treated area. Use only lukewarm water for bathing the area.

- Use an electric shaver if you must shave the treated area, but only after checking with your doctor or nurse. Do not use preshave lotions or hair removal products on the treated area.

- Protect the treatment area from the sun. Do not apply sunscreens just before a radiation treatment. If possible, cover treated skin with light clothing before going outside. Ask your doctor if you should use a sunscreen or a sunblocking product.

If so, select one with a protection factor of at least 15 and reapply it often. Ask your doctor or nurse how long after your treatments are completed you should continue to protect the treated skin from sunlight.

- If you have questions, ask your doctor or nurse. They are the only ones who can properly advise you about your treatment, its side effects, home care, and any other medical concerns you may have.

These recommendations can improve your quality of life while electing to do chemotherapy/radiotherapy and facilitate the healing process. The above recommendations are consistent with the National Cancer Institute.

The Journey Toward Healing

The road is hard, the journey swift
As we travel towards the grave.
This body will return to dust
But what of the soul to save?

Healing is a journey involving our spirit and soul; without their involvement, the body cannot heal.

The Road to Healing

When we experience pain, most of us want immediate relief. However, there are deeper pains that lodge within us and fester over time causing more devastating illness, including the loss of hope and spiritual death. Total healing is not just relief from physical suffering. Even when we continue to suffer from physical ailments, we can experience healing on a soul and spiritual level. Medical science tells us there are many incurable diseases, including cancer. Most of these diseases kill the body. However, medical science does not deal with the diseases of the spirit and soul—the very essence of life.

Where are we to turn when we are given crushing news about our health? The natural human tendency is to react rather than respond. When diagnosed with cancer, we often react with fear instead of responding in faith. Cancer is an illness that can steal the essence of life and breed a hopelessness that takes away the life of the soul and spirit. I have many patients who are fighting cancer. I have very few patients who give up. The key word is to fight. Life is worth the battle against a potentially fatal illness. But how do we fight? To whom do we turn when our defenses are weak?

And fear not them which kill the body, but are not able to kill the soul. —Matthew 10:28

We must turn to the supernatural existence of God. We must reach out to God and ask for His divine intervention through prayer and diligent search. We must search for the answers He gives through His Word (the Holy Bible) and the guidance He gives through others whom we trust, whether it is family, a friend, a physician, or a clergyman. God gives life and He gives it abundantly! When we take the steps allowing God to bring healing to our innermost being, we can have the assurance that the final outcome is an excellent one.

Which Path To Follow?

Believe that life is worth living and your belief will help create the fact. —William James

To be healed from sickness and disease, we must focus on the precious gift of life. We must turn away from our old patterns of living and be transformed into a new existence. This transformation will include life-giving fruits, such as love, peace, joy, kindness, and faith. We must have faith! In the King James version of the Bible, Jesus says: *"For verily I say unto you, That whosoever shall say unto this mountain, Be thou removed, and be thou cast into the sea; and shall not doubt in his heart, but shall believe that those things which he saith shall come to pass; he shall have whatsoever he saith"* (Mark 11:23). Faith is believing that we will possess what we hope for. Faith healing is not superstition nor is it accomplished through the efforts of a single person. Healing comes from God and God alone.

There is a woman mentioned in the Bible who had a bleeding disorder for many years. She had gone to many physicians and was helped by none of them. She said, "If I may touch but his clothes, I shall be whole" (Mark 5:25-28, KJV). She persisted until she saw herself well. What a powerful example of faith. The key is to believe in the source of all-perfect healing—God Himself.

There are many healers in our day and age. Many of them draw from powers that are dark and oppressive. I call these types pseudo-healers (false healers). My friends, this type of healing is temporary and may last for a moment of time. However, the healing that comes from God is for all eternity and there are no negative effects associated with it. Latch on to the power of God and cry out to Him for your complete healing. Trust Him, for He is able to do more than we could ever expect.

The Best Source of Medicine

Looking to medical science alone for answers to our deepest needs is a waste of precious life energy. The very best source of medicine comes from God's Word. In Proverbs 4:20-22, the Scripture tells us that the words spoken from the mouth of God are life-giving. Reading and growing in God's Word is the best medicine any of us can get. This doesn't mean that we discard the best that traditional and alternative medicine have to offer. The Word of God will help us to know what is the best course for our healing. What action would be appropriate and have the best outcome? How do I proceed? When we are diligent students of His Word, we learn wisdom and we gain understanding. The Holy Spirit gives us guidance and keeps us from potential harm. Not only is our faith in His healing ability made stronger, but our understanding deepens and we develop prudence in our decision making. The Word of God is the first source of medicine.

Prayer: The Best Defense

Our healing is not only a journey, but a battle. In the Book of Job, we have a clear illustration of the battle that is waged for our very existence. This battle for life must be fought with powerful weapons. Prayer is the most essential weapon we have. God is our only true source of life, and He alone has the power over it. God is aware of the battle; and through prayer, we liberate His power to defeat the unseen forces of evil. He goes to battle for us! He did battle for Job! Read the Book of Job. It is an intriguing account of God's power, deliverance, and healing.

It is essential in prayer to remember that through His name the battle is won. In and of ourselves, we are powerless. We must do all we can, but the power to overcome belongs to God; and when we rely upon Him, we find deliverance from the oppressive forces of sickness and disease. Our prayers do not have to be complicated dissertations, but rather, simple words of faith.

We can pray simply with faith by saying:

"Oh God, provide Your complete healing and deliverance from this affliction and restore me physically, emotionally, and spiritually. Facilitate Your healing energy within my body, and renew every cell and body system through the name and power of Jesus Christ and the power of His blood. Cause me to grow in my soul and spirit. Restore this worn out body with Your renewed body. Cause me to rely upon Your judgment and complete will for my life. I leave my life in Your hands and trust that the essence of my life is secure with You. In Your trusted and sacred name. Amen."

Finally, realize that it is essential for you to know God on a personal level. Before you can understand His power fully, you must accept Him in your heart completely. Jesus said, *"If ye abide in me, and my words abide in you, ye shall ask what ye will, and it shall be done unto you"* (John 15:7, KJV). We must know that Jesus died so we may live. In order to know Him, we must denounce our old way of living and accept His saving grace and become a follower of His way to the end of our human existence. His power is available for your healing.

May God bless and heal you completely in body, soul, and spirit and may your life be filled with peace, joy, and hope until His coming.

Amen!

Where the Rubber Meets the Road

May God guide you, your loved ones, and your doctor to the appropriate, integrated treatment of cancer with the greatest result.

W here the rubber meets the road is when a cancer patient experiences remission and cure. Yes, there are numerous accounts of people beating the odds of cancer. The following four cases are real experiences but the names have been changed to protect privacy and confidentiality.

Breast Cancer

Lisa is a 50-year-old female who was diagnosed with breast cancer by her regular physician. She came to my office hoping that alternative medicine could help her. After much discussion, she decided to implement the suggested treatment plan. Fortunately, her cancer had not spread to other areas of her body. Her treatment plan consisted of the following:

- Intravenous immunotherapy (includes vitamins, minerals, amino acids, immune modulators)
- IP-6

- MGN 3
- Beta 1,3-Glucan
- Larix
- CoQ10
- Selected Chinese botanicals
- Hoxsey formula
- B12, folic acid, and B comp injections 1-2 times weekly
- Multivitamin/mineral formula
- Adrenal support
- UltraClear Plus, along with dietary guidelines
- Juicing
- Probiotics

Lisa also had several chemotherapy sessions which consisted of Taxatera, Taxol, and Adriamycin. She is in complete remission.

Lung Cancer with Spread to the Brain

Joanne, 45 years old, came to my office after consulting many alternative practitioners. She was frustrated because she was on confusing regimens and feeling discouraged because her cancer was getting worse. Her diagnosis was lung cancer. She was having seizures when she came to see me. Joanne was a smoker and consumed moderate amounts of alcohol. She was told that she was going to die within the month because the cancer had spread to her brain and liver. I started Joanne on a comprehensive regimen and told her that she needed to work with an oncologist who was open to the alternatives. She agreed. I referred her to an oncologist whom I work closely with. The following regimen kept Joanne alive for three years:

- Intravenous immunotherapy (vitamins, minerals, amino acids, and immune modulators)

- MGN 3
- Beta 1,3-Glucan
- Larix
- Hoxsey formula
- CoQ10
- B12, folic acid, and B comp injections 2 times weekly
- Essiac formula
- Selected Chinese anti-tumor botanicals
- Dietary changes which included cutting out red meats and juicing every day
- IP-6
- Several chemotherapy sessions (standard regimen for lung cancer)

The response to the regimen was excellent. After three months of therapy, we repeated MRI to see if the cancer was clearing. MRI results demonstrated no brain lesions and liver metastasis was gone and the size of the lung lesion that was previously grapefruit-size had shrunk to about the size of a golf ball. Joanne was so happy that she felt she didn't need to continue such a strict treatment regimen and eventually her office visits became less frequent to none. Joanne and I had an ongoing battle with her smoking. I told her that she needed to quit or the cancer would return. She didn't take the advice. About one year later, I received a call from Joanne and she had a desperate tone. She said, "My cancer has returned! Can you please help me?" I told her I would. This time she stopped smoking. I put her on the same regimen and stepped up the frequency of her visits. Again, her cancer responded to treatment. But she began smoking again, and the cancer returned. She lived for three years, even though her doctors told her that she only had one month. This case makes me sad when I think of the many more years she could have had . . . if she had just stopped smoking.

Prostate Cancer

Dave is a 62-year-old retired 747 captain. He is in great physical shape except for the fact that he was just diagnosed with prostate cancer. He had a high PSA and a significant Gleason score. His biopsy demonstrated cancer confined to the prostate gland with no spread. He came to me by a referral, and he heard about the good things that were happening with the cancer patients that I have had opportunity to treat. I started him on a treatment regimen that consisted of:

- IP-6
- PC SPES
- Beta 1,3-Glucan
- B12, folic acid, and B comp injections 1-2 times weekly
- CoQ10
- Vitamin E
- Concentrated Saw palmetto extract
- Multivitamin/mineral/antioxidant formula
- Dietary changes which included intense juicing

Dave's PSA levels dramatically reduced to the normal range and allowed for the entrance into a treatment program that used proton therapy that rated a high cure rate for prostate cancer. We achieved excellent results with the alternative regimen, and Dave was happy. He wanted to be sure that the cancer was cured so he enrolled in the proton treatment program at Loma Linda, and we continued supportive care. He made it through the treatment, and he is cancer-free and healthy!

Multiple Myeloma

Susan is a 55-year-old female who came to see me after being diagnosed with multiple myeloma. She had heard the devastating stories of people who suffered with this form of cancer. She wanted to do everything she could from an alternative perspective that was safe and effective. She had one round of chemotherapy, and this made her very ill. She stopped and told me that she needed to do something naturally. I designed a program for her to follow:

- IP-6
- Beta 1, 3-Glucan
- MGN 3
- B 12, folic acid, and B comp injections 2 times weekly
- Dietary changes including juicing
- CoQ10
- Hoxsey formula
- Essiac formula
- Probiotics
- Selected Chinese botanicals with anti-tumor and immune modulating properties
- Immune enhancing therapy
- Stress reduction

Susan didn't need any more chemotherapy. She is currently in a steady state with no flare-up of the myeloma. This is going on three years from the time of the diagnosis. She is very happy.

There are many more cases like these that include lymphoma, leukemia, testicular cancer, and sarcomas. The common theme of all these cases is that life was extended and the quality of life improved. In addition, there is even the hope of being cured. There is also another vital element in all of these cases that I must tell you about, and that is prayer. In every case that comes, I pray for guidance and prudence in developing a plan. In addition, I petition God, on my patient's behalf, asking that He would cause the cancer to remit and, if it is His will, to be cured. I mention specifically that cancer cells with their genetic traits would die and healthy cells would develop free from all cancer. In my opinion, the credit for the healing in these cases belongs to God! May He also guide you, your loved ones, and your doctor to the best integrated approach to cancer with the greatest result.

Conclusions and Cancer Resources

Integrating the best treatment options available is the key to healing. Some treatments are known to be curative and some are experimental. It is necessary to be informed as to the treatments available and when to integrate treatments.

This book is compiled to give you, the health-conscious individual, more information so you can make a better health care choice. When it comes to cancer, you need to know. God bless your healing journey.

Testing Resources

AMAS: ONCOLAB, 36 The Fenway, Boston, MA 02215. 1.800.922.8378

CBC: Carbon Based Corporation. 1.702.832.8485

ELISA/ACT: Serammune Physicians Lab. 1.800.553.5472

ION and Oxidative Protection Panel: MetaMetrix, Inc., 5000 Peachtree Ind. Blvd., Norcross, GA 30071. 1.800.221.4640; www.metametrix.com

Product Resource Information

Antineoplastons - Burzynski Clinic. 713.335.5697; www.cancermed.com

Issels' Vaccine (also known as autologous vaccine) - 1.888.4ISSELS or 1.888.447.7357 from USA and Canada; www.issels.com

Chelation Therapy - www.chelation.com and www.ehealthandhealing.com

Larix is available from Eclectic Institute at 1.800.332.4372

Iscador is available from Waleda at 1.800.241.1030.

Viscum album (homeopathic mistletoe extract) is available from Biological Homeopathic Industries (BHI) at 1.800.621.7644.

For professional name brand herbal and nutritional products, contact Emerson Ecologics at www.emersonecologics.com or 1.800.654.4432.

For information on PC SPES, contact Dr. John A. Catanzaro, Health&Wellness Institute, 5603 230th St. S.W., Mountlake Terrace, WA 98043, (425.697.6112) or read *The Best Options for Diagnosing and Treating Prostate Cancer* by James Lewis Jr., Ph.D. (ISBN 1-883257-04-2) and *The Herbal Remedy for Prostate Cancer* by James Lewis Jr., Ph.D. (ISBN 1-883257-02-6).

Cancer Resources

National Cancer Institute Information Resources

You may want more information for yourself, your family, and your doctor. The following National Cancer Institute (NCI) services are available to help you.

Cancer Information Service (CIS)

Provides accurate, up-to-date information on cancer to patients and their families, health professionals, and the general public. Information specialists translate the latest scientific information into understandable language and respond in English, Spanish, or on TTY equipment.

> Toll-free: 1.800.4-CANCER (1.800.422.6237)
> TTY: 1.800.332.8615

The Center of Integrated Medicine (CHIPSA)

CHIPSA is a progressive healing center that focuses upon the whole person. At CHIPSA, prayer and compassionate care are the cornerstones of healing. Here is an excerpt from their web page:

The human body is truly one of God's most amazing and complex creations. The many systems that make up our bodies participate in a wonderfully integrated relationship that we have labeled "life." Among the most amazing systems of the body is the immune system. It is the powerful tool that keeps us healthy and disease-free. The condition and functionality of the immune system is the primary factor in the body's fight against all diseases.

The physicians of the Center of Integrated Medicine believe that many of today's "incurable diseases" are in many cases "incurable" due to the limitations of the approach of traditional medicine to only attack the local manifestations of a disease. They believe that in order to heal the body of disease, medicine must concentrate on the body as a whole and the insufficiencies in the various body systems, especially the immune system. They have observed and treated patients with many of these diseases successfully. Of course, each patient is unique and must be evaluated individually for the proper approach to a possible solution.

Visit CHIPSA at www.chipsa.com

Internet Information

Health&Wellness Institute

5603 230th St. S.W.
Mountlake Terrace, WA 98043
1.425.697.6112
www.ehealthand7healing.com

American Cancer Society

1599 Clifton Road, N.E.
Atlanta, GA 30329-4251
1.800.ACS.2345
www.cancer.org

Cancer Research Institute

681 Fifth Avenue
New York, NY 10022-4209
1.800.33.CANCER
www.cancerresearch.org

Cancer Care, Inc.

1180 Avenue of the Americas
New York, NY 10036
1.800.813.HOPE
www.cancercareinc.org

The Candlelighters Childhood Cancer Foundation

7910 Woodmont Ave., #460
Bethesda, MD 20814-3015
1.800.366.2223
www.candlelighters.org

Cancer Research Foundation of America

200 Daingerfield Road, #200
Alexandria, VA 22314
1.800.227.CRFA
www.preventcancer.org

National Cancer Institute

31 Center Drive/MSC 2580
Building 31, Room 10A07
Bethesda, MD 20892-2580
1.800.4.CANCER
www.nci.nih.gov

Additional Internet Sites

www.cancerhelp.net

www.searchforcures.com

www.phrma.org (listing of the latest cancer research drugs)

www.cancermed.com

www.chipsa.com

www.issels.com

cancernet.nci.nih.gov

www.chelation.com

www.metametrix.com

www.llu.edu

For more information contact:

Health&Wellness Institute, Inc.
5603 - 230th Street S.W.
Mountlake Terrace, WA 98043
www.ehealthandhealing.com

For book orders contact:
1.800.862.4811

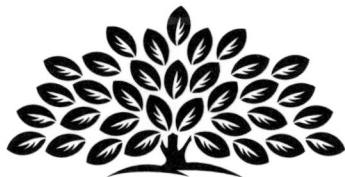

Health&Healing Press_{TM}

Index

A

abdominal
    cancer 40
    pain 91
accine 148
acemannan 90
acetaminophen 101, 104
acid/alkaline diet 85
acid-base balance (pH) 30
acidophilus 74–75
adrenal support formula 88
Adriamycin 142
aflatoxins 18
AIDS 46, 96
ajoene 100
alcohol 17, 23, 37, 63, 105,
    122, 142
alimentary canal 98
alkaline 85
alkaloids 93, 97, 101
alkamides 95
allergies 21, 36, 51
allicin/alliin 99
aloe vera 90–91
aloe-emodin 90
aloin A/B 90

alpha carotene 72
aluminum poisoning 98
alveolar foci 54
AMAS 29, 38
AMAS-ONCOLAB 147
amino acids 33, 35, 65, 69,
    71, 88, 91, 141–142
amygdalin 91
anemia 75, 108, 127
anesthesiologist 125
anesthetic, general 30–31
anger 126
animal research 49–50, 67,
    90, 93, 95, 100, 103,
    105, 108
anthraquinone tabebuin 107
anthrone-10-C-glykosyls 90
antibiotics 21, 75, 104
antibody 44–45, 49, 87, 99,
    132
    human antimouse
        (HAMA) 50
    production 33, 55
    radiolabeled 132
    therapy 51
anticoagulant 100–101, 108
antigen 38, 41–42, 44, 49–
    50, 132
antimony trisulfide 104

antineoplastons 56
antioxidant 19, 34, 36–37, 76, 87, 102, 144
antiseptic washes 105
anxiety disorders 104
apigenin 102
apoptosis 110
appendicitis 91
appetite 83, 98, 121
    loss of 69, 92
arabinogalactans (larix) 91
arsenic 16, 20
    sulfide 105
arthritis 52, 92
aspartame 18
aspirin 101, 104
asthma 52
astracylodes 109
astragalus (astragalus membranaceus) 91–92, 109
astraglycosides I-VII 91
atherosclerosis 36, 103
ATP 36
autohemolysates 55
autoimmune disease 96
autonomous nervous system 56

B

B cells (B lymphocytes) 44, 46, 50
bacterial vaccines 52
bad breath 103
basal cell
    skin cancer 26
    types 18
beta carotene 37, 72
Beta-1 3 D-Glucan 77
betatrons 130
bifidus 75
bioaccumulation 22
bioflavonoid 106
biological
    response modifiers (BRMs) 45
    terrain assessment (BTA) 30
    therapy 43–45, 50–51, 111–112
biopsy 31, 35, 144
    prostate 38
biotherapy 43
birth control 20, 61
birth defects 103
black tea 102, 104
bladder 98, 119
    cancer of 23

burdock root (arctium
lappa) 99, 105
burns 90

C

cadmium 20, 37
caffeine 17, 101, 103, 122–
123
withdrawal 104
Caisse, Rene 97
calcium 64, 72, 105
cancer
acceleration of 17
causes of 16–24
costs 28
definition 15
detection 26, 29–42
resources 147–148
risk 15, 17–20, 24–25,
29, 63, 74, 102
survival rate 25–26
vaccine 52, 54, 148
candida 84
car fumes 57
carbohydrate metabolism
74
carbonated drinks 105
carcinogenesis 107

carcinogenic substances 57
carcinoma
in situ 26
cardiac ischemia 36
cardiotoxicity 105
carotenoids 72
cascara 105
case study
breast cancer 141
lung cancer 142
myeloma 144
prostate cancer 144
cat's claw (uncaria
tomentosa, uncaria
guianensis) 93–94
catalase 37
catheter 116
CBC 31, 147
central nervous system
problems 128
cerebral ischemia 36
cervical cancer 24, 38, 72,
131
Chace, Daniella 79
Chaitow, Leon ND, DO 65,
68
chelation therapy 20, 22,
33, 65–69, 148
chemo/hormone therapy 54

cryptosporidium 23
curcumin 103
cyclamates 18
cyclosporine 94, 97
CYP 2E1(enzyme) 101
CYP 3A4 (enzyme) 97
cytogenetic studies 30
cytokines 44–47
cytotoxic action 132

D

D'Adamo, Peter 85, 91
dairy foods 86
deficiencies
    nutritional 16–17, 71
    potassium 90
degenerative disease 52–53
dehydration 105
depression 126, 128
dermatitis 101
desserts 84
detoxification 20–22, 53,
    55, 65, 77, 81, 87, 98,
    106
DHEA 63, 88
DiaBeta 101
diabetes 34, 84, 107
diagnosis 27
diarrhea 92, 97, 105, 108

diary 122
diet 2, 21, 33–34, 63, 143–
    145
    acid/alkaline 85
    Blood Type 85
    deficiencies 17
    food-combining 85
    Mediterranean 99
    therapy 71, 78–87
    vegetarian 86
digestive 33, 109
    imbalance 16
    symptoms 66
    tract 85, 119
        cancer 102
        problems 51
digital rectal exam 42
dihydroxyanthraquinones
    90
diuretic 90, 93
diverticulitis 93
dizziness 108, 127
DNA 37, 73–74
dressing, flax-seed oil 83
drugs
    antiarhythmic 90
    anticancer 49–50
    antinausea 122
    cardiac 90

chelating effects 68
chemotherapy 113, 123
conventional 21
cortisone-like 94
immune-suppressive 16,
21
pharmaceutical 89
toxicity 36
dysentery 92

E

echinacea 94–96
Eclectic Institute 91, 148
eczema 95
edema 80
EDTA chelation 66–68
Ehrlich ascites tumor 68
electrolyte imbalance 105
electron beams 40
ELISA/ACT 20, 32, 147
endogenous factors 55
end-stage pathology 37
enema 82, 128
coffee 82
enzyme 41, 74, 77, 80, 84,
101
digestive 33
protein 37
therapy 55

epigallocatechin-3-gallate
(EGCG) 102
epigen 127
epithelial 55
Epstein-Barr virus 24
erythropoetin 127
esophagus 73, 119
essiac herbs 97–99, 143,
145
estrogen 59
fractionated 63
medications 60, 62
receptor (ER) 60–62
replacement 60
excretory system 53
exogenous factors 55
extracorporal zone 55

F

family cancer syndrome 19
fat 17, 34, 63, 73–74, 81,
97–98
"bad" 34
"good" 34, 74
hydrogenated 34
trans fats 34
fatigue 20, 33, 66, 72, 86,
92, 118, 121, 127–128,
134

fatty
    acids (EFAs) 17, 34, 64, 74
    cells 22
    deposits, arterial 97
    toxins 98
fear 138
Fecal Occult Blood Test 42
feet, cold 20
fever 51–52, 133
    therapy 55–56
fibrinolytic action 100
fillings 33
first-degree family history 25
fish 17, 34, 72, 74, 85, 102, 129
flavonoids 90–91, 97, 102
flaxseed 34, 74, 83
flu 128–129
fluorine 23
foci
    alveolar 54
    dental 54
    head 54, 56
    tonsillar 54
folic acid 73, 75–76, 88, 142–145
folk medicine 93

food
    additives 16, 18
    organic 84
    preparation 83
    processed 17–18, 34
    smoked 17
    whole 19
free radical 16, 19, 34, 36, 66, 76–77, 87, 102
    activity 34, 37
    chain propagation effect 37
    damage 34
    definition 19
    pathology 36–37
Fu Zhen therapy 109
fungus 107

G

gallbladder 106
gamma rays 131
ganoderma 109
garlic 73, 86, 96, 99–101
gastritis 93
gastrointestinal 74, 87
G-CSF (colony-stimulating factor) 48
germanium 73, 99
Gerson 74, 79–80, 83, 85
    meals 84

Mexican hospital 81
Therapy Handbook 81
Giardia 23
ginseng 88, 109–110
gland
    adrenal 87–88
    pituitary 87
    prostate 144
    reproductive 87
    thymus 99
    thyroid 87–88
glandular system 87
Gleason score 38, 144
glucose 72
Glucotrol 101
glutathione 19, 86
glutathione peroxidase 37
glycoside 95
GM-CSF (colony-
    stimulating factor) 48
gonorrhea 92
Grave's disease 52
green tea 101–103
gum tissues 66

H
hair 34
    analysis 20, 32
    follicles 119
    loss 75, 125–126, 132

HAMA (human antimouse
    antibodies) 50
hands, cold 20
headache 20, 66, 104, 123
Health&Wellness Institute
    3, 32, 105, 151–152
heart 74, 97, 100, 119
    attack 100
    disease 26, 34
    pounding 127
    rate 93, 102, 104
    rhythm 104
hematologist 30
hematopoietic growth
    factors 48
hemoccult 33
hemorrhage 97, 108
hemorrhoids 93, 128
hepatitis B virus (HBV) 24
hepatitus C 24
herbal
    preparations 134
    therapy 89–110
herbal therapy 63
herbicides 16, 22
herbs 21, 63, 76, 89–110
herpes simplex 95
heterocyclic amines 102

high linear energy transfer
(high LET) radiation
131
hip 30
Hippocrates Soup 81
Hismanal 97
HIV (human
immunodeficiency
virus) 24
homeostasis 110
homeostatic function 55
hopelessness 137–138
hormonal
analysis 20
balance 63, 88, 110
dysfunction 16, 63
imbalances 20
system 53
hormone 17, 26, 41, 61
female 102
receptor assay 35, 59
replacement therapy
59–63
soy-based 62
therapy, natural 21
hormone-related cancer 74
Hoxsey formula 104, 142–
143, 145

HPV (human
papillomavirus) 24
HTLV-I (human T cell
leukemia/lymphoma
virus-I) 24
hybridoma 49–50
hydration 17
hydroxyaloins 90
hydroxytoluene 19
hyperpyrexia 55
hyperthermia 52, 54, 132
hypoxic conditions 37

I

immune
activity 75, 108, 110
cells 44
defense 19, 21, 45
function 67, 69, 72, 76–
77, 101
modulating 77–78, 92,
141–142, 145
reactivity 32
regulation 21
response 17, 21, 32, 44–
47, 50, 91, 96
stimulation 78, 91, 105
suppression 32, 72, 77

monocytes 45
mouth 119
   cancer of 24
   sores 123
MSH2 (gene) 20
multiple sclerosis 96
mushroom extract
   maitake 107
   shiitake 107
mutations 19, 25, 103
myeloma 47, 144–145
   case study 144
myricetin 102

N

naphthoquinone lapachol
   107
National Cancer Institute
   (NCI) 26, 43, 51, 130,
   135, 149, 151
nausea 105, 108, 118, 120,
   122
neck, cancer of 40
nerve transmission 33
nervous system 75, 98, 119
nervousness 104
neupogen (colony
   stimulating factor) 128

neural
   disturbance 55
   system 53
   therapy 55
neuroblastoma 50
niacin 76
nickel 20, 33
night sweats 92
Nizoral 97
Noroxin 104
nutritional
   deficiency 17, 71
   factors 17
   glandular support 87
   imbalance 17
   replacement 63, 65, 120
      IV 69, 120
   replacement therapy 69,
      71–78
   supplementation 71
   support therapy 120

O

oncogene 16, 22, 57
oncologist 30, 61, 111, 125,
   130, 142
organic acids 34
organic food wash 86
organisms, infectious 16

ovarian cancer 47, 59
oxidation 30, 34, 36–37, 76,
    100, 103
oxygen 73–74, 98, 127
    chain-terminating 37
    therapy 55

P

Panadol 101
pancreas 23, 98
pantothenic acid 76, 88
Pap smear 38, 42
Papanicolaou, George 38
Parafon Forte
    (chlorzoxazone) 101
pathology
    end-stage 37
    free radical 36–37
pau d'arco (tabebuia
    impetiginosa, tabebuia
    avellanedae) 108
Pauling, Linus 76
PC SPES 40, 109–110, 144,
    148
pectin 108
pelvic 39
    cancer 40
    examination 42
Penetrex 104

peptides 57
periodontitis 103
peroxidation, serum lipid
    36–37
pesticides 16, 22, 36–37
pH (acid-base balance) 30
phagocytosis 45, 55
pharmacist 124
phosphonates 30
photon radiation 130–131
phytochemical 73, 84
phytohormonal properties
    63
Phytopharmica's Cellular
    Forté (IP-6) 77
plasma cells 44
platelets 48, 103, 133
Plavix 101
Plendil 97
pneumonia shot 129
poisoning 98
    aluminum 98
    lead 98
    mercury 98
    metal 66
polio vaccine 129
polyphenols 103
    catechins 102

polyporus umbellatus (Jian Pi Yi Qi Li Shui) 109
polysaccharides 91
postmenopausal women 60–62
potassium 74, 80, 84, 98
    deficiency 90
    iodide 105
pregnancy 91, 94, 104, 108
premenopausal women 61
preservatives, food 19
prickly ash bark 105
proanthocyanadins 19
probiotics 74–75, 142, 145
Procardia 97
Propulsid 97
prostate 39, 109
    cancer of 24, 28–29, 38–40, 51–52, 144
    case study 40, 144
    enlargement 38
    exam 42
    inflammation 38
    ultrasound 38
prostatitis 95
protein powder 86
proteins 33, 44, 71, 85, 132
proton therapy 40, 144

PSA (prostate-specific antigen) 38–39, 42, 144
psoriasis 95

Q

quercetin 102
quinone compounds 107
quinovic acid glycosides 93

R

radiation 19, 40, 46, 48, 52–54, 56–57, 75, 98, 102, 121, 130
    conventional 40
    damage 132
    exposure 30, 132
    external 131
    high linear energy transfer (high LET) 131
    ionizing 37, 130
    photon 130
    therapy 43, 50, 111–113, 130–133
radioimmunotherapy 132
radioisotopes 50
radiolabeled antibodies 132

radionuclide 30
radioprotectors 131
radiosensitizers 131
radiotherapy 111, 130, 135
  external beam 130
  internal 131
  research 132
  side effects 132–133
radium 131
rashes 51
rectum
  cancer of 24
regional lymph node
  involvement (N) 28
relaxation exercises 124
remission 27, 52, 56, 86,
  97, 141–142
renal cell 47, 51
  carcinoma 46
respiratory
  distress syndrome 36
  tract infection 95
reticulo-histiocytary zone
  55
reverse osmosis 23
rheumatic diseases 36
rheumatism 92, 107
riboflavin 76

RNA 37, 73–74

S

saliva 20, 30, 63, 123
sarcoma 46, 52, 109, 145
saw palmetto 64, 110, 144
screening-accessible
  cancers 24
selenium 19, 75, 99
Serammune Physicians Lab
  32
serum lipid
  peroxidation 37
sheep sorrel (rumex
  acetosella) 99
shortness of breath 127
sigmoidoscopy 42
silybum marianum (milk
  thistle) 106
silymarin 106
Sjoegren's syndrome 52
skin 34
  cancer of 18, 24, 130
  color 132
  irritation 132
sleep, loss of 121
slippery elm bark (ulmus
  fulva) 99

particle beam radiation
131
proton 40, 144
radiation 43, 46, 48, 50,
52–54, 56, 75, 111–
113, 121, 130–133
radioimmunotherapy
132
radiotherapy 111, 130–
132, 134–135
TNF (tumor necrosis
factor) 48
thiamin 76
thiazide diuretics 90
throat 23, 92, 123
thymus gland 99
thyroid 34, 72
thyroid support formula 88
Ticlid 101
tiredness 51, 132
tissue damage syndrome 80
tissue rejection 21
TNF (tumor necrosis factor)
therapy 48
TNM staging system 27
tongue, cancer of 23, 130–
131
tonsillar foci 54
toxicity
alcohol 37

cadmium 37
cigarette smoke 37
drug 36
intestinal 16
ionizing radiation 37
lead 37, 67
metal 16, 20, 32, 36, 66
pesticides 36–37
solvents 36
trace
mineral 73–74, 84, 92,
99
nutrient 72, 75
transplantation 21, 30, 50
triterpene
glycosides 91
tuberculosis 96, 99
tumor 18, 24, 27, 35, 45,
47–48, 50–51, 53, 60–
62, 64, 67–68, 73–74,
78, 80–81, 90–91, 100,
103, 105, 107–110, 112,
130–131, 143, 145
benign 99
brain, benign 40
inoperable 56
malignant 53
markers 35, 41

necrosis factor (TNF)
46, 48, 103
operable 56
remission 56
vaccines 50, 52
tumor-associated antigens
41
tumor-milieu 53
tumor-suppressor genes 57
turkey rhubarb root (rheum
palmatum) 99
Tylenol 101

U

ubiquinone 72
ulcerative colitis 91
ulcers 92–93, 104, 107–108
ultrasound 35, 63
prostate 38
ultraviolet radiation (UV-B)
103
uña de gato (cat's claw) 92–
93
uncaria guianensis (cat's
claw) 92
uncaria tomentosa (cat's
claw) 92
uranium 131
urinary
analysis 20, 33

bladder 26
cancer of 102
infection 95
urine 30, 63, 66
uterine
cancer 59, 131
cervical cancer 130
uterus 20, 52
UV filtration 23
UV rays 18

V

vaccinations 21, 46, 51–52
vaccine
bacterial 52
cancer 54
chicken pox 129
Issels' 52, 148
live virus 129
mycoplasma 52
pneumonia 129
polio 129
tumor 50, 52
vegetables 72, 76, 82–83,
85–86
soup 81
Viagra 97
vinegar 83, 105
viral infections 94
viruses 16, 21, 24, 93, 95

vitamin 63, 65, 68–69, 75–
    76, 84, 88, 101, 141–
    142, 144
    A 19, 37, 72, 95
    antioxidant 34
    B complex 75–76
    B12 75–76, 88, 142–145
    B17 91
    B6 75
    C 19, 37, 63, 76, 87, 95,
        105
    E 19, 37, 63, 76, 87, 95
    K 108
vomiting 105, 108, 118,
    122

W

water 17, 22, 73, 77, 129
    polluted 16
    salt 80
    softener 80
weight 55, 63
    gain 84
    loss 84, 87
    maintenance 87

X

x-ray 30–31, 35, 40, 98,
    130–131

Y

yeast 77, 107
    tablets 105

Z

zinc 77, 88, 96
    chloride 104
Zocor 97

About the Authors

Dr. John A. Catanzaro, president and founder of the Health&Wellness Institute, is a naturopathic physician who received his education and training at Bastyr University, America's leading university in alternative medicine. He maintains a private practice in Seattle. Along with being a health care consultant and member of the Washington Association of Naturopathic Physicians, Dr. Catanzaro is an author, lecturer, and ordained minister.

Elizabeth Chapin is a freelance writer, wife, and mother of four. She received her degree in Communication and began a technical writing career in the Silicon Valley. Since moving to the Northwest, she has worked on a variety of projects, from educational curriculum to public relations materials.